430528

Fitness

Through

Aerobics & Step Training

Karen S. Mazzeo, M.Ed.

Morton Publishing Company
925 West Kenyon Avenue, Unit 12
Englewood, Colorado 80110

Cover Design by Bob Schram, Bookends, Inc., Boulder, Colorado

Editing by Carolyn Acheson, Modesto, California

Typography by Ash Street Typecrafters, Inc., Denver, Colorado

Illustrations by Susan Strawn, Loveland, Colorado

Cover Photo and Interior Photography by Jeffrey Hall Photography, Haskins, Ohio

Acknowledgments

Special appreciation is extended to the following individuals who have shared their time and superior talents in this endeavor:

Laura Ware Babbitt
Robert E. Baird
Stephen I. Block
Richard W. Bowers
Philip H. Goldstein
Jeffrey Hall
Peter Holmes
Virnette D. House
Carin Peirce Johnson
Marian Larkin

Lauren Mangili
Lisa Mark
Katherine Marwede
Mary Beth Mazzeo
Douglas N. Morton
Peggy Paul, R.D., L.D.
Bernard Rabin
Carrie A. Robinson
Sue Schoonover

Appreciation is given to the following for granting permission to use copyrighted materials:

Kenneth Cooper, M.D., M.P.H., and Bantam/Doubleday/Dell .
National Dairy Council and Oregon Dairy Council
Werner W. K. Hoeger, Ph.D., and Morton Publishing Company

A special thank you to the following companies by providing apparel and equipment with which to photograph:

Nike, Inc., One Bowerman Drive, Beaverton, OR 97005 (1-800-535-6453) for women's fitness apparel

Mark Cooksey, Manager, Foot Locker, Bowling Green Mall (Ohio) (419-354-0567) for Nike Aerobic and Reebok Cross-Trainer Shoes

Sports Step, Inc., for The Step and instructional videos. For additional information, call Sports Step, Inc. (1-800-SAY-STEP)

SPRI Products, Inc., 1554 Barclay Blvd., Buffalo Grove, IL 60089 (1-800-222-7774) for rubber resistance bands and tubing, and men's SPRI shirts.

Dedication

To Peter Holmes and Mary Beth Mazzeo
the cover smiles and physiques of
Fitness Through Aerobics & Step Training.
May the start of each of your career-goal dreams come true this year.
You are two very talented, special people!

Table of Contents

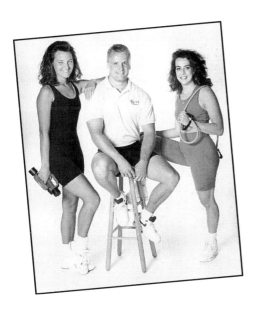

Introduction

This book details and illustrates the latest fitness research available. It assists individuals like yourself, who are taking courses in physical fitness, to understand the principles and techniques involved in aerobic exercise-dance and step training and also how to structure a complete physical and mental training program that will work for you for a lifetime.

The two fitness activities just mentioned — aerobic exercise-dance (also called aerobics) and step training (which uses a 4–12″ step bench) — are two of the most popular current methods for achieving and maintaining physical fitness. Aerobics has enjoyed two decades of unbelievable success, and step training, although a relatively new activity, is rapidly attaining the same highly acclaimed distinction as THE way to fitness.

Fitness Through Aerobics and Step Training is an abridged version of my latest text, *Aerobics— The Way To Fitness*. Both have been developed for fitness course enthusiasts to fill the dual needs that aerobics and step training present. This abridged text, however, is designed primarily for the novice needing just the basics. Its brief, easy-to-follow, sequential learning order can be the map and compass for your journey toward personal excellence, providing the methods for how to achieve your total fitness goals.

To strongly encourage taking the action of beginning and committing to a *Fitness* program, Chapter 1 introduces the mental training concept of *anchoring* the fitness mindset. This refers to understanding how *to solidly blueprint (anchor) the best fitness choices so you are able to <u>make</u> the best fitness choices — anywhere, all day, every day.* Anchoring a fitness mindset *occurs* when we are feeling strong feelings and whatever is happening around us, consistently at the moment, gets linked up to it (see Introduction opening photo). Understanding the mindset process, what makes up the self-management model, and how to use each for a permanent and positive change, is described in the opening chapter.

Chapter 2 provides definitions for terminologies used and provides the foundation from which to build the physical fitness techniques you will choose to use.

Chapter 3 gets your program underway by establishing where you are today through testing procedures that enable you to describe your starting point. From there, you can choose your goals, and you will have the ability to monitor your progress and see your results.

Chapters 4 and 5 present the basic building blocks, the principles, for developing your own aerobics and step training programs. The four segments of each program are described in Chapter 4. To add variety to the aerobics or step training and strength training segments of your program, ideas on how to perform interval aerobics, combining both, are suggested in Chapter 5.

All physical fitness programs must be built upon a foundation of safety and on the needs and concerns that arise both from a preventive standpoint and after-the-fact. Chapter 6 first lists possible program challenges or problem areas and then solutions to consider. It emphasizes proper body positioning (posture), because good positioning, especially of the spine and joints, underlies all physical movement you will ever choose to do. This chapter is, therefore, paramount, and where the techniques of your physical fitness program must begin.

Chapter 7 presents techniques you can use in your segments from start to finish, illustrated by numerous photographs. Included are: (a) basic

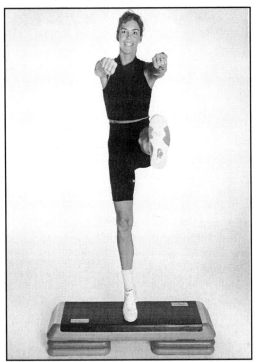

Figure I.1. Stepping up onto the bench, taking weight on your **left** foot, kick your **right** leg forward, waist-high.

aerobics steps and gestures for each of the four program phases; (b) the six basic bench approaches and basic step training patterns, including several popular variations; and (c) techniques for using rubber elastic bands and tubing, and hand-held weights, alone or in conjunction with the bench.

The exercise movements are all described and then photographed using a "mirrored" method. A movement described and visualized as using the left foot/arm/or side of the body is actually the right foot/arm/side of the model (see Figure I.1). Thus, you do not have to reverse the direction of what is pictured and what is performed. You simply perform the movement on the same side of the body as you see it photographed and described.

Chapter 8 takes apart the *how to* of both aerobics and step training choreography, for planning on your part. You'll find unlimited possibilities for using a variety of movement.

Chapter 9 presents the principles of stress management and follows with relaxation techniques. Understanding creative ways to rejuvenate your mental and physical energy immediately following exercise is the revitalizing touch needed for the final segment of the physical fitness workout.

Complementing all of the information on exercise and energy expenditure is Chapter 10, which focuses on the intake of energy — your diet and current nutritional concerns. Weight management strategies follow, in Chapter 11, as a basis for a healthy and natural slimness.

The text concludes with Chapter 12, which presents you with the option to rank your fitness priorities and to establish total program goals toward which to strive.

For your convenience, an index of key topics is also included.

■   ■   ■

You are the master of your ship.
Nothing, and no one else,
can do it for you.

■   ■   ■

Student Information Profile

Please fill in the following information, remove from the textbook, and give to your instructor:

Name _____Rank: F/So/J/S/Grad/Other

Address _____Phone _____

Social Security No._____Age_____Height _____Weight _____Ideal Weight _____

Rate Your Fitness Level   **SUPERIOR/EXCELLENT/GOOD/**FAIR/POOR/VERY POOR—PRE

SUPERIOR/EXCELLENT/GOOD/FAIR/POOR/VERY POOR—POST

Previous class or instruction in course: _____

Sports in which you participate/enjoy weekly: _____

Reason(s) for taking course: _____

Did anyone recommend this course or instructor? _____

If so, whom? _____

Physical limitations _____

Activity that you would especially like instructor to cover: _____

Heart rate: Resting_____Training Zone _____– _____

List any drug you take (which may alter your heart rate): _____

Do you desire to: (circle) Gain lean weight / Lose fat weight / Stay same

Do you smoke? _____If so, number per day:_____

Rate your alcohol consumption: Never/Daily/Other/ _____

List interest in music, favorite song, favorite artist:_____

Other interests_____

If 45 or older or have specific limitation: I have my doctor's written permission to participate.

Doctor's name and phone: _____

I have read and understand the responsibilities for participants and the instructor.

_____   _____
Signature   Date

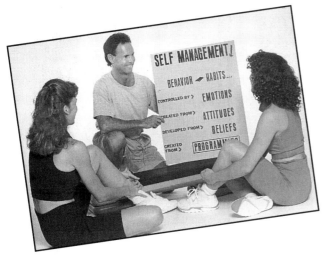

1

Anchoring a Fitness Mindset

To develop a mindset for the fitness lifestyle, we must first become more aware of the choices we constantly make and what internal resources we have used to make these choices. We, and others around us, can experience directly the choices we make. We can clearly see, hear, and feel these responses. What we usually can't immediately detect is *how* — what process — led us to those choices. Therefore, if we begin to consider the factors underlying our actions — the emotional forces, attitudes, beliefs, and programming already present and operating our "mental computers" — we can then understand fitness for a lifetime and have it become the programmed belief (*mindset*) we consistently choose.

First we must recognize the steps of the fascinating process we go through, in a split second, when we are faced with an immediate fitness choice in our daily lifestyle. ("Shall we take the stairs or ride the elevator up the two flights to the classroom today?") Taking the process apart, step by step, helps us to know where our mindset needs repair and allows us to change and insert new constructive possibilities. Let's begin this journey by taking a look at the self-management model[1] that identifies the underlying factors fueling and influencing our choices (as shown in the chapter opening photo), and then establishing how to anchor a consistent fitness mindset.

BECOMING AWARE OF YOUR CHOICES: BEHAVIORS/ ACTIONS/HABITS

Whatever we call it — behavior, actions, or habits — our choices are the end result of a unique problem-solving strategy we have within ourselves. A problem-solving strategy consists of how we perceive, store, and retrieve information about something. We initiate this problem-solving strategy by bringing the outside world inside us so we can interpret it. We do this by using our three predominant senses: visual (sight), auditory (hearing), and kinesthetic (bodily sensations, such as touch and muscle movements). To a much lesser degree we use our remaining two senses of taste and smell.

We blend these external sensory stimuli with the internal sensory stimuli stored inside of us. These internal resources include pictures or images (visual), self-talk (the auditory dialogue we constantly say to ourselves about what's going on), and emotions (kinesthetic, internal body sensations).

As an example of the individual steps of the mindset process: You go to the fitness facility you've joined. You see two exercise classes going on simultaneously in rooms side by side (external visual stimuli) and hear the background music accompanying each class (external auditory stimuli). Both are using familiar exercise steps and gestures (external kinesthetic stimuli) you enjoy (an emotion, which is an internally felt kinesthetic stimuli). One workout session consists of a new activity you've never seen or done before, using a bench/step piece of equipment (you have no visual/auditory/kinesthetic stimuli resources because you've never seen, heard, or felt it). The other is a familiar aerobic dance-exercise class you've experienced many times (you have internal and external visual/auditory/kinesthetic resources). The choice to join either session is yours.

Your problem-solving mechanism will be processing possible solutions to this question in split-seconds, through self-talk dialogue similar to one of the following. Do you see, hear, and feel yourself in any of these solutions?

- ■ "I enjoy the exercise-dance class (kinesthetic, emotions) and know the routines (kinesthetic, muscle movements). I don't feel (kinesthetic, emotions) like thinking about (processing new visual images, auditory sounds, and kinesthetic movements) and trying the new bench/step class right now."

- ■ "I feel so clumsy today (kinesthetic, both feelings and muscle movements) that I know I'd slip (kinesthetic, muscle movements, and maybe visual pictures or auditory sounds) on the bench/step. I don't want or feel (kinesthetic, emotions) like having this new challenge (using all my senses to build resources) after the day I've had today!"

- ■ "Wow! I can do that (am willing to engage all three senses)! With a little direction (in developing new visual and auditory stimuli) on how and where to begin moving (kinesthetic,

muscle movements), I'll have a new, fun, exciting choice to bring variety into my fitness-for-life program."

■ ■ ■

How you will problem-solve the fitness choices you make (or ANY choices you will ever make, for that matter!) will come from your own internal thoughts — visual pictures you're making to yourself, auditory stimuli of external words and sounds or internal dialogue you're saying to yourself, and kinesthetic stimuli or body sensations you're experiencing or choosing to experience.

■ ■ ■

The lifestyle choices you make are, therefore, not made for you by someone or something else. *Your choices occur within you*, in that beautiful mental computer called your mind. "Because thought results in behavior immediately, the only control that is ever needed is thought control, and that entails only my present willingness."[2] The first step toward understanding how to make healthy fitness choices is becoming aware of all of the resources available for us to use, both externally and internally.

You will next recognize that external stimuli are available to all of us and that we all have the ability to create helpful internal stimuli that can lead to good choices. We must, however, filter out all the stimuli (both external and internal) that do not seem relevant at the moment to the problem at hand and focus only on what will fulfill our present, or most valued, wants or needs. (Again, this happens in fractions of seconds of time.) We complete this mindset process with a response: our *choice*!

How do we each uniquely filter the multitude of sensory resources available to us and come up with poor or healthy choices? That key lies in dissecting the remainder of the self-management model. Clarifying what directly precedes our choices is the next step in this looking-inward process (Figure 1.1).

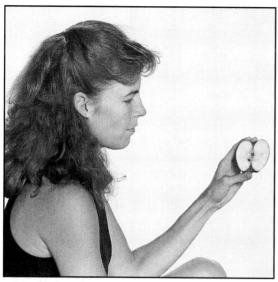

Figure 1.1. Like dissecting layers of an apple and looking deeper within, we will come to the center, the core, the programmed seed — understanding how we make the choices we do.

THE EMOTIONAL FORCES THAT DIRECT AND CONTROL OUR CHOICES

We each have an innate survival mechanism within us that strongly encourages us to avoid pain and to gain pleasure. (The various emotions that make up the all-encompassing categories of pain and pleasure will be discussed more specifically in Chapter 9, to enable you to experience, in depth, the *re-linking* process that will occur when a fitness challenge perceived as painful becomes a pleasure.)

The dual forces of pain avoidance and pleasure gratification are at work while we are problem-solving the challenges we face. For example, do we refuse the magnificent, high-calorie dessert our hostess has made especially for us (emotional pain) and stick to our firm commitment to ourselves to completely eliminate high-calorie/low-nutrient desserts from our diet intake? Or do we say "yes" (emotional pleasure)

for whatever rationalized reasoning we come up with at the moment?

Problem-solving anything in our lives usually consists of trying to remove the problem (pain) as quickly as possible so that feeling good (pleasure) can again be ours (Figure 1.2). We often are not willing to endure the emotional pain that all self-discipline, growth, and change seems to require. We might say to ourselves, "Do I really have to do all these abdominal crunches every day (pain of waiting for the gratifying results) to have a tight, toned abdomen, or is there a shortcut (to the pleasure of having the results)? I hate strength training (pain, either emotional or physical). Maybe if I just don't eat as many sweets, my abdomen will get smaller and look toned (instant pleasure gratification)."

The desire for pleasure is always the end result of *any* goal we have. This may seem like common sense, but the ramifications of what is said here can have profound impact on your ability to make healthful choices.

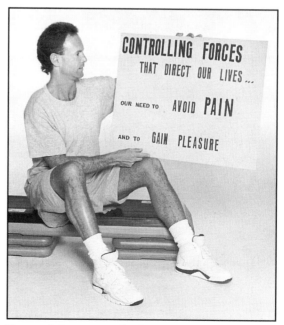

Figure 1.2. Pain is the force we want to get rid of quickly so we can experience the joy of feeling good.

■ ■ ■

A key to making and continuing a fitness commitment is to learn to accept delayed gratification (immediately having the results you desire long-range) and develop the growth and discipline (enduring the pain — delaying of immediate gratification) required for change — permanent, blueprinted change — to occur.

■ ■ ■

What determines whether we are directed and controlled by the force of pleasure and immediate gratification or whether we can accept the pain of delaying instant gratification regarding the choices we make? What creates the willingness to endure waiting for growth and change to happen?

YOUR ATTITUDE

The third step involved in the self-management development process entails examining our attitude. "The way we see things shapes the kinds of experiences we have . . . Our attitudes are truly the lenses of the mind through which we perceive reality. . . . Up in your head and mine are thousands of these attitudes . . . They are capable of making the same given experience either pleasant or painful."[3]

Your attitude — that perspective or lens of positive and negative, open and closed-mindedness, and the enabling and disabling dispositions you take — is the true reflection of the opinion you have about something. When asked, most individuals say they have an overall positive attitude, but you need only to monitor your attitude for several days to realize how difficult it can be to maintain a positive outlook on life's many challenges.

Statistics from the medical and communication fields tell us that more than 75% of all we experience is negative.[4] From the radio/TV/news media to all the other stimuli we encounter, the volume of negative input we see, hear and feel vastly outweighs the positive. The challenge to develop and keep a positive, open mindset is tremendous. It takes a willingness and dedication to actively and continuously choose it.

Choosing to establish or keep an open, positive mindset as a lifestyle is made possible by becoming keenly aware of your attitude toward problems and challenges you experience in your everyday living. One of the ways you can do this is to listen and monitor — by writing down — your *self-talk*. Self-talk represents numerous ways to speak *to* yourself, out loud and silently within; and *about* yourself to others, out loud and in written and taped form.

We talk to ourselves 100% of our waking hours, about everything we're experiencing — seeing, hearing, emotionally feeling and physically touching, tasting, and smelling. Observing your own self-talk will be a real eye-opener and will generate the awareness you need to more quickly achieve some of the goals you'll soon set. You will observe that negative self-talk is said or recorded using past and future tense verbs. Positive self-talk is stated and recorded in the present tense, using verbs ending in *ing*, creating the feeling that the present action is happening now.

In addition to self-talk, a second clear indicator of your attitude is experienced through your kinesthetic sense — *your physiologies and how you move*. For example, "When exercising . . . if you work hard and you're short of breath and you keep saying to yourself how tired you are or how far you've run, you will indulge in a physiology-like panting or sitting down that supports that communication. If, however, even though you're out of breath, you consciously stand upright and direct your breathing into a normal rate, you will feel recovered in a matter of moments."[5]

A third indicator of your attitude may at first be rather abstract to experience or "see" for the novice, but with awareness and practice it can be as powerful as your self-talk and physiological expressions. It involves the *mental images or pictures you make*, how close/far away, color/black-and-white, moving/still, they are, and whether you are in the images (associated) or removed from the images and are observing (disassociated). A vast amount of exciting research is going on with all three of these factors that influence attitude, and thus, one's health and fitness. The body of information called *neurolinguistic programming*, or NLP, and the relatively new science of *psychoneuroimmunology* are both good resources to look into if you desire more information on the topic.[6]

> Studies in neuroscience and psychobiology have shown that the way you think can affect your body and its performance. For example, stressful events perceived as threatening produce hormones in the body that reduce exercise efficiency and increase fatigue. However, when a stressful situation is viewed in a more positive light, as a challenge rather than a threat, other chemicals . . . are released in the body, producing improved exercise performance.[7]

Once you are aware of how powerfully the factors that make up your attitude affect your adherence to a fitness program, it will become an exciting challenge to do something constructive to improve them to bring about the changes you desire. It will be motivating to develop repetitive, positive self-talk (called *affirmations*), enabling physiologies (more effective postures and breathing techniques), and positive images (which are more colorful, close up, and active) that you are now choosing to hear, feel, and see about yourself and your program. "If you are consistently delivering congruent messages to your nervous system that say you *can* do something, they signal your brain to produce the result you desire, and that opens up the possibility for it."[8]

The key thought with attitude is openness — saying, picturing, and feeling "I can" and then remaining open for the answer to *how*. Your brain will continually search for possibilities when the channels and pathways are kept open.

Clearly, your attitude is paramount to having a mindset for successful, healthy living. But you will immediately become aware that just *telling* yourself positive affirmation statements, or *visualizing* helpful images, or engaging in various

motivational movements regarding goals you would like to achieve (and actually *achieving* the goals) can be two separate phenomena — if your search for solutions stops there. It doesn't.

What does determine your ability to color an experience or perspective positively or negatively? What is responsible for developing your attitudes and cementing them permanently, for adherence and consistency? It's time to go one step deeper within and take a look at *what lies at the foundation of the entire mindset process*. What seed lies at the core of our choices?

YOUR BELIEFS: THE KEY TO UNDERSTANDING YOUR PROGRAMMING

Whether you call them guiding principles, rules for living, faith, philosophies for life, or truths you value, your beliefs ultimately determine the behavioral choices you make. Some of the beliefs we hold originated from an intensely significant experience (one in which all of our senses were *vividly* involved) and some, over time, by a collection of less intense experiences. What are beliefs? Here are a few definitions to ponder:

- useful thoughts that can provide meaning and direction in life.

- statements that we have accepted as the truth and are useful, given to us by all the significant people in our life that we trust: parents, grandparents, pastors/rabbis/priests, relatives, brothers and sisters, peers, teachers, coaches, advisors, specific media sources, and so on.

- pre-arranged, organized filters to our perceptions of the world.

- commanders of the brain, which deliver a direct command to our nervous system.

- the compass and maps that guide us toward our goals.

What is remarkable is that we continually make choices based on the programmed beliefs we have and value, and many times these beliefs are old, worn out hand-me-downs that we have accepted and never really questioned for personal validity. You are now in a maturing process within your life's journey, where intellectual growth is expected along with physical development, so you must be sure the beliefs you are following concerning fitness and developing a healthy mindset are the best around. There is no universal rule stating that old, worn out, programmed beliefs can't be changed. Life *is* change and growth and involves stretching one's self to the limits of his or her own potential.

People who have significantly changed history are those who have greatly changed our beliefs. Think about that, then realize that your beliefs can really help you to change an unwanted behavior, especially if you have some key new beliefs that work, are useful, and do not infringe upon the wants and needs of others.

Ponder each of these beliefs that are extremely helpful when considering a positive change in your fitness mindset:

> *"This moment is a fresh, new opportunity. The past does not equal the future."*
>
> Tony Robbins

> *"The only definition for 'failure' is when I stop trying something altogether. I've reprogrammed all other ideas of failure (when I don't get what I wanted or needed) to mean I've just received 'feedback' / 'results'."*

Take a moment now and begin to establish a collection of beliefs you have about living a healthy lifestyle. Continue listing helpful beliefs throughout your fitness course. Stating, picturing, and feeling yourself believing these thoughts will assist you in blueprinting the fitness-for-life mindset.

SELF-MANAGEMENT OVERVIEW

Immediately preceding or underlying our choices are our emotions, attitudes, and beliefs. This last resource we have stored within, our beliefs, constitutes our ultimate valued guidelines for living that we have fully accepted and allowed to become programmed onto our own "mental tapes." *If we are to change our choices, we ultimately must update our disabling, no longer useful beliefs.*

The change process does not have to take a long time. Begin to more closely observe behavior, emotions, attitudes, and beliefs of present-day people who are successful role models of excellence and who exemplify the fitness lifestyle you would like to have. By duplicating their positive strategies, you will gain a shortcut toward achieving your own mindset for fitness. You will soon begin to realize that all healthy lifestyle choices or strategies are like time-honored recipes. They contain key ingredients, in defined measureable amounts, used in a prescribed order for consistently good results.

ANCHORING A FITNESS MINDSET

You've made the decision to adopt an all new, healthy lifestyle choice. *When you begin to consistently feel strong, positive feelings about it* because you've used positive emotions, attitudes, and beliefs to make that choice, a solidly programmed *link* will be made and it will be securely "anchored" into your thinking process.

Reinforcing this link, or anchor, through repetition will more permanently solidify your newly blueprinted choice. You can achieve this by actually physically repeating the fitness choice or through mental training — rehearsing the choice through audiotapes, imaging, and other means. *Change is a choice!*

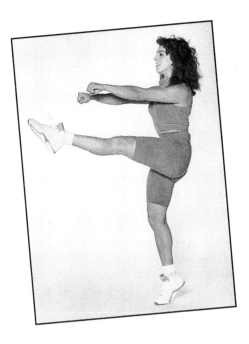

2

Aerobic Exercise: A Key To The Fitness Lifestyle

Consider these two familiar philosophies: "Use it or lose it!" and "Knowledge is power." Both represent powerful beliefs that can put to the test the mindset for the fitness lifestyle you are now developing.

The first belief — "Use it or lose it" — can be applied to all the dimensions of your physical wellness and must rank at the top of the priority list of choices when it comes to achieving and maintaining a physically healthy lifestyle. The second belief — "Knowledge is power" — sounds good but requires updating before it can become a belief that actually works for us. Knowledge of all the fitness benefits and test results is not enough to change a sedentary mindset or improve one's total physical fitness. *Actions* must be combined with all this knowledge. Updating the latter belief to state, "The application of knowledge is power" is a completed thought and will enable us to get moving.

COMBINING MENTAL CONDITIONING WITH PHYSICAL FITNESS

Get Motivated

In beginning the journey toward physical fitness through participation in aerobics (dance-exercise), don't just sit back and absorb the many ideas coming your way through this text and course. Think creatively: "How can I use each point of knowledge as it comes to me?"

By immediately developing powerful images, internal self-talk, and emotion-filled movements, you will be more likely to retain the information and solidly blueprint it so more information can be added later. These three key elements — powerful images, internal self-talk and emotion-filled movements — are the basic building blocks of the abstract thought we call *motivation!*

Get Ready, Get Set . . .
The Researched Findings

Our mental approach to the physical fitness challenge has been established. We are armed with the knowledge of how to become motivated, and we are *ready*! Now we can *set* the stage and solidify — with reason, facts, and statistics — why we should go for it all and become physically fit.

Physical conditioning through an activity such as aerobics will assure you a happier, more vivacious and abundant life. And the physically fit active lifestyle actually prolongs life.[1] Furthermore, "Some predictions are that by the end of this century, the average American woman will live to age ninety, and the average American man to the mid-eighties.[2] With these impressive findings and a projected long life ahead of us, let's make sure it will be a *quality* long life we're living (not just doing time), by making good choices.

Aerobic/Aerobics/Aerobic Dance-Exercise

Most simply stated, the term *aerobic* is an adjective that means *promoting the supply and use of oxygen*. The body's demand for oxygen increases when you engage in vigorous activity that produces specific beneficial changes in the body. Aerobic can, therefore, refer to *any type of exercise mode as long as certain basic criteria are met*.

Within the last decade the exercise mode entitled *aerobic dance*, or more generalized to the term *aerobic exercise*, has been abbreviated and hyphenated to the currently popular terms *aerobics* or *aerobic dance-exercise*. Throughout this text, and in the professional journals of today, these terms are used interchangeably to mean the same activity. So keep the distinction: *aerobic* is an adjective describing another word, and *aerobics* is a noun denoting a mode of activity.

Healthy Lifestyle Choices

Associated regular fitness behaviors that enhance the ability to perform well during physical conditioning workouts include eating nutritionally, maintaining proper body weight, relaxing, and getting an adequate amount of sleep. Without a balance in *biochemical functioning* — energy intake, energy expenditure, and energy rejuvenation — the effects and benefits mentioned later will not occur. Each of these healthy lifestyle choices is introduced here, and expanded in later chapters.

Eating

To provide the fuel needed to produce the energy required for all aerobic exercise, and to insure proper body regulatory functions, growth, and repair, participants should eat a well-balanced diet that provides all the nutrients needed to stay well, to be able to perform well, and to maintain a proper weight.

Regarding how much to eat and the time of day for eating, food intake should follow a *25-50-25 rule*: 25% of intake for breakfast, 50% for lunch, and 25% for the evening meal. Incidentally, weight control is easier for those who exercise either before breakfast or one and one-half hours after the heaviest meal of the day.[3]

For greatest efficiency, participants should refrain from eating for one, or preferably two, hours before participating in aerobic activity and, instead, eat afterward. In digesting food, an increased amount of blood and oxygen is needed in the digestive tract. With exercise, as much as 100 times more oxygen is needed in the working muscles (arms and legs) than when at rest. The body has great difficulty increasing blood and oxygen to two major body functions at once.

Relaxing and Sleeping

Quality time should be set aside for reflective relaxation and adequate sleep. These are important restorative mechanisms. Aerobics takes a great deal of energy, and the body's way of restoring energy is through relaxation and sleep, which help restore the ability to concentrate and to maintain a positive attitude. Physiologically, relaxation and sleep help by lowering both the body temperature and the heart rate, which, in turn, lower the body's demand for oxygen and nutrients, thereby conserving while restoring the body's supply of energy.

A Total Physical Fitness Conditioning Program

Total physical fitness is the positive state of well-being allowing you enough strength and energy to participate in a full, active lifestyle of your choice. It is "the general capacity to adapt favorably to physical effort. Individuals are physically fit when they are able to meet both the usual and unusual demands of daily life, safely and effectively without undue stress or exhaustion," according to the American Medical Association.

A total physical fitness conditioning program consists of five basic parts. This can be visualized by the fitness triangle, depicting three action-type components, centered around two underlying structural components, as shown in Figure 2.1.

1. *Aerobic fitness* (cardiovascular and respiratory)
2. *Flexibility* (ability to bend and stretch)
3. *Muscular strength and muscular endurance* (thickening muscle fiber mass to enable individuals to endure a heavier work load)
4. *Good posture* (holding body in proper position for safety and efficiency)
5. *Body composition* (maintaining proper fat weight to lean weight ratio).

Aerobic Fitness

A total, well-rounded weekly fitness conditioning program should consist of regular participation in all five components. Because the sign of genuine fitness is the condition of the heart, blood vessels, and lungs, however, aerobic fitness is the most important component. By engaging in aerobic dance-exercise, or any other aerobic activity (such as the currently popular step-training), the heart gradually strengthens and develops a greater capacity to pump more oxygenated blood to the body with fewer contractions. Exercised hearts are stronger and slower.

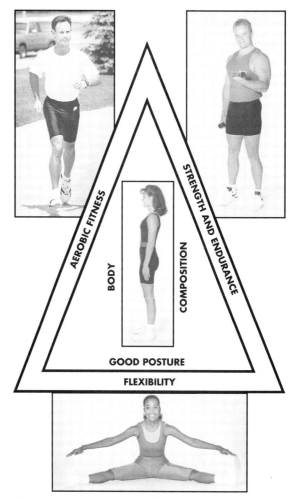

Figure 2.1. Fitness triangle.

Highly trained and conditioned endurance athletes have resting heart rates as low as 30 to 32 beats per minute, an unbelievably low rate! What actually happens is that with regular, stimulating exercise, the heart becomes a more efficient pump. It pumps more blood with each stroke, and with a more efficient stroke volume, your heart can function with less effort. By getting your heart into condition, you may be practicing preventive medicine. You may be lessening the danger of a coronary heart attack, five, ten, fifteen, twenty years from now. And if you do have one, your chances of surviving are far greater with a heart, lungs, and blood vessels which are in good condition.[4]

A person can exist without big, bulging muscles, or without the perfect figure, or with a head cold, but not very long without a good heart and lungs. Unfortunately, more than 40 percent of all people who have a first heart attack do not receive a second chance to change their habits or develop an aerobic program; they die.[5] And more than half of all American deaths each year are attributable to heart-related diseases.[6] If only we could establish a living pattern priority early in life to counteract this overwhelming statistic!

Flexibility

Flexibility is defined as the functional range of motion of a certain joint and its corresponding muscle groups. The greater the range of movement, the more the muscles, tendons and ligaments can flex or bend. Muscles are arranged in pairs. One muscle's ability to shorten or contract is directly related to the opposing muscle's length or stretch. Flexibility is maintained or increased by movement patterns that slowly and progressively stretch the muscle beyond its relaxed length. The stretch is performed to a point where tension developing in the muscle is felt, but not to a point of pain.

Muscular Strength/Muscular Endurance

Muscular strength is the ability of a muscle to exert a force against a resistance. Strength activities increase the amount of force that muscles can exert, or the amount of work that muscles can perform. Activities such as weight training can develop strength in the skeletal muscles.

Muscular endurance is the ability of muscles to work strenuously for progressively longer periods without fatigue. It is the capacity of a muscle to exert a force repeatedly, or to hold a static (still) contraction over time.

Muscular strength and endurance activities do not provide increased oxygen to condition the heart to function more efficiently.[7] Their primary target is skeletal muscle.

Good Posture/Good Positioning

Proper positioning of the body when performing any type of physical exertion promotes a safe and efficient workout. Once the basic mechanics are known and practiced, this underlying fitness component becomes an integral part of every move, not a separate program.

Body Composition

An individual's total body weight is composed of fat weight and lean weight (fat-free weight). Keeping an appropriate percentage ratio between these two weights is important for the entire body's best functioning and helps prevent the onset of obesity and its many related health risks. This fitness component is managed by establishing a proper diet and exercise plan that provides for ideal weight maintenance.

If you aren't beginning your program at your ideal weight, specific guidelines will be given within both the physical exercise programs and the dietary eating plans you'll establish for how to achieve your ideal percentage ratio.

In summation, of the five components involved in developing a total physical fitness conditioning workout program (your *prescription exercise plan*), aerobic fitness training is considered the most important. The remainder of this chapter is devoted to a detailed look at the research and general principles recommended for you to follow, including modes of activity you choose and the individual techniques you use. The other four physical fitness components are more fully explained in later chapters.

AEROBIC FITNESS TRAINING

Aerobic Capacity Improvement: Your Main Objective

Aerobic means promoting the supply and use of oxygen, and *training* refers to muscle stimulation. Therefore, aerobic training is any exercise that requires a steady supply of oxygen for an extended time and demands an uninterrupted work output from the muscles.

Activities such as aerobic dance-exercise and step-training significantly increase the oxygen supply to all body parts, including the heart and lungs, through continuous, rhythmic movement of large muscles and connective tissue. This type of movement conditions the body's oxygen transport system (heart, lungs, blood, and blood vessels) to process the use of oxygen more efficiently. This *efficiency in processing oxygen* is called *aerobic capacity* and is dependent on your ability to:

■ Rapidly breathe large amounts of air.

■ Forcefully deliver large volumes of blood.

■ Effectively deliver oxygen to all parts of the body.

In short, one's aerobic capacity depends upon efficient lungs, a powerful heart, and a good vascular system. Because it reflects the conditions of these vital organs, *aerobic capacity is the best index (single measure) of overall physical fitness*.[8]

Aerobic capacity is what is measured, quantified, and labeled in a physical fitness stress test, performed either in a laboratory (called a laboratory stress test) or on a pre-measured distance such as a track (called a field stress test). You are given the opportunity to test your aerobic capacity in Chapter 3, using either method.

Strengthening The Heart: Progressive Overload Principle

Aerobic dance-exercise, step-training, or any aerobic activity conditions the heart muscle by strengthening it through a principle called *progressive overload*. Not only will the heart pump more blood with each beat, but it will also have longer rests between each beat, thereby lowering the pulse rate. Aerobic exercise overloads the heart by causing it to beat faster during a specific time-frame of the workout session, making a temporary high demand on the cardiorespiratory system. Over time, as you become more fit, the heart eventually adjusts to this temporary high demand, and soon it is able to do the same amount of work with less effort.

By *overloading* the heart with any vigorous aerobic exercise, your aerobic capacity increases and a desirable training effect can be achieved. The *training effect*, or total beneficial changes that usually occur, consists of:

■ Stronger heart, sending more oxygenated blood to all tissues of the body.

■ More blood cells produced.

■ Slower resting heart rate.

■ Expansion of blood vessels.

■ Improvement of muscle tone.

■ Lower blood pressure through improved circulation.

■ Stronger respiratory muscles.

■ Regulation of the release of adrenalin.

■ Increased lung capacity.

■ More regular elimination of solid wastes.

■ Lower levels of fat found in blood,[9]

■ Strengthening of muscles and skeleton to protect them from injury later in life.

■ Deterring osteoporosis by increasing bone density.[10]

■ Increased sensitivity to insulin and lowered blood sugar levels in mild, adult-onset diabetes.[11]

■ Improvement in the way the body handles cholesterol, by increasing the proportion of blood cholesterol attached to high-density lipoprotein — a carrier molecule that keeps cholesterol from damaging artery walls.[12]

Aerobic Exercise Alternatives

Aerobic exercise options include all of the following activities:

■ Aerobic dance-exercise (aerobics)

■ Bench/step-training

■ Cross-country skiing

■ Cycling (including stationary cycling)

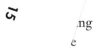

...ng
...e

- Ska... e/roller/in-line)
- Stair climbing
- Swimming
- Walking/hiking (moderate to fast pace-walk).

Aerobic Criteria

These exercise alternatives, collectively, have several essential criteria for the exercise to be labeled *aerobic* (see Figure 2.2). Because *aerobic* means *with oxygen*, the movement that you do must:

1. *Use the large muscles of the body*,[13] (your arms and legs). Exercise gesture and step patterns found in aerobic dance-exercise and bench-step movements are excellent choices.

2. *Be rhythmic.*[14] One-two-one-two, using a steady beat of music, with either a fast or slow tempo, is suggested.

3. *Practice a minimum of three sessions per week.*[15]

- Four days a week or every other day is good.

- Some key researchers recommend five days as a maximum for fitness goals. Beyond this, injuries to the musculoskeletal system from overuse are ten times more likely to occur. Give your body at least two days off per week, especially if you are a novice to physical fitness conditioning.

- If your goals are related to more than just aerobic fitness — if, perhaps, your profession (e.g., fitness instructor) or your athletic sport status requires more workouts or days per week — allow your body to tell you your maximum frequency. A sudden elevated resting heart rate in the morning

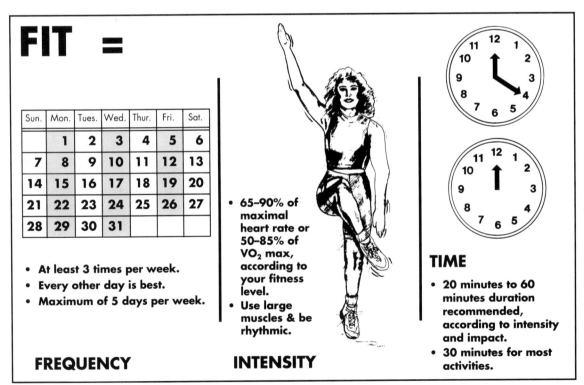

Figure 2.2. Five aerobic criteria.

signifies the day(s) not to work out. This is your built-in body signal, and it can be readily seen/heard/felt simply by daily monitoring your resting heart rate. Upon arising in the morning, check this heart rate for one full minute.

4. *Exercise continuously for 20–60 minutes.*[16]

   ■ Duration depends upon the intensity and the impact of the activity. (Both of these terms are explained later in full detail.)

   ■ Lower intensity activity, such as walking, should be done over a longer period (40–60 minutes).

   ■ Because high-impact types of activity, such as running and jumping, generally cause significantly more debilitating injuries to exercisers, shorter workouts (20 minutes) are recommended.

5. To receive the cardiorespiratory fitness benefits (called the training effect), *the heart rate must be maintained in a specific target heart rate training zone*, which is the individualized safe pace at which to aerobically work or exercise. This reflects your intensity and is explained scientifically as one of the following:

   ■ 65–90 percent of your maximum heart rate or

   ■ 50–85 percent of your maximum oxygen uptake, or heart rate reserve.[17]

Intensity Detailed

Frequency and time duration of your workouts are easy to determine but the amount of exertion during the workout to keep it safe while continually making fitness gains can be more of a challenge to determine, especially for the novice. Intensity is measured or monitored in one of three ways:

■ Finding your target heart rate (THR) training zone using the Karvonen formula. This is suggested for the novice.

■ Using the psychophysical scale for ratings of perceived exertion (RPE), which shows a high correlation with heart rate and other metabolic parameters according to American College of Sports Medicine (ACSM) guidelines. Rate of perceived exertion monitoring is suggested for the individual who already has become well-accustomed to taking a heart rate pulse.

■ Using the talk test. This easy and practical method is best used in conjunction with the THR and RPE for monitoring exercise intensity.

Your Target Heart Rate Training Zone

Taking Your Pulse

To calculate appropriate exercise intensity using this method, you first must know how to accurately take your pulse. The pulse equals heartbeats per minute and can be felt and counted at one of six pulsation points. Select which area you can best obtain a pulse using your index and second fingers. The two places most often used to count pulse are the neck near the carotid artery and the wrist near the radial artery. Both are shown in Figure 2.3.

1. The carotid artery, located in the neck, is usually easy to find. Place your index and middle fingers below the point of your jawbone and slide downward an inch or so, pressing lightly. When you use the carotid artery pulse-monitoring method, make sure to apply light pressure, as excessive pressure may cause the heart rate to slow down by a reflex action.

2. The radial artery extends up the wrist on the thumb side. Place your index and middle fingers just below the base of your thumb. Press lightly. Count the number of pulsations, or beats, for 60 seconds. The total is the number of heartbeats per minute. To count correctly, make sure you count each beat you feel.

Having gained the skill of pulse taking, it is now time to establish your *resting heart rate*. This number is to be placed in the formula for establishing your target heart rate training zone.

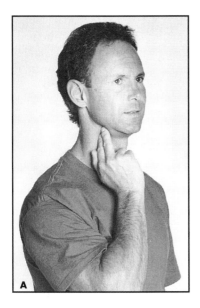

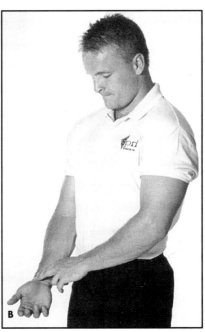

Figure 2.3. Taking the carotid pulse (a) and the radial pulse (b).

One of the two visible signs of improvement in heart and lung fitness is a lower resting heart rate. Because the RsHR is the basic thermometer of fitness, after a ten-to-fifteen-week aerobics course, you and your classmates may experience:

■ An average –3 heartbeats per minute resting heart rate decline.

■ An average –10 heartbeats per minute by smokers who quit (or significantly change their consumption) during the course and as much as a –24 heartbeats per minute decline.[18]

Monitoring the Resting Pulse Rate

A true *resting heart rate* (RsHR) is not taken in a class but, instead, when the individual has been at complete rest, preferably, sleeping for several hours and upon awakening. Keep a clock or watch with a second hand next to your bed. When you awaken (without an alarm clock ring), take your pulse for one full minute and record that number as your RsHR. Do this for five consecutive mornings, then determine an average (add all RsHR's and divide by 5). This is a rather accurate determination of your resting heart rate.

NOTE: *Unusual stress and illness (illness is a type of stress) sharply elevate the resting heart rate from previous readings.*

Normally healthy individuals should, therefore, find a positive outlet for stress. It (stress) affects you even as you sleep (constant rapid heart rate), a time when the heart ideally should take a break and slow down for six to eight hours.

Determining Your Target Heart Rate Training Zone

Your average RsHR figure is now placed in the formula for determining your target heart rate training zone. The other variables figured into the formula are current *age* and *lifestyle*, represented as a percentage of maximum heart rate.

If you are:	Use:
■ a non-athletic adult	50% to begin
■ sedentary	60–69%
■ moderately active	70–75%
■ very active and well-trained	80–85%

Record your age and the selected percentage range from above that describes your lifestyle. Figure the Karvonen equation. The result is your target heart rate, the safe exercise training zone for you.

How to Figure Your Target Heart Rate Training Zone

Since three basic factors enter into figuring your estimated safe exercise zone, those must be established first:

1. Your current age:_____

2. How active is your life-style? _____% MHR. If you are:
    (Choose one:)
    - Non-athletic adult: use 50% of your maximum heart rate.
    - Sedentary: use the figure 60–69% of your maximum heart rate
      (but only for the first two or three weeks).
    - Moderately physically active: use 70-75% of your maximum heart rate.
    - Active & well-trained: use 80-85% of your maximum heart rate.

3. Your average resting heart rate: _____

Now place your numbers in the formula that follows:

A. 220   – _____ = _____ **Estimated Maximal Heart Rate (MHR)**
    (Index number)   (Your Age)

B. _____ – _____ = _____
    MHR   **Resting HR**   **HR Reserve**

C. _____ × . _____ = _____ + **Resting H.R. =** _____ *
    Heart Rate Reserve   Lower end life-style activity range   R
    (i.e. #2 above)   A
                                                                                             N
    _____ × . _____ = _____ + **Resting H.R. =** _____ * G
    Heart Rate Reserve   Higher end life-style activity range   E
    (i.e. #2 above)

RANGE OF _____   * This range is your estimated safe exercise zone. Keep your
YOUR   heart rate working in this range while you aerobically exercise for
TARGET   _____   * approximately 30 minutes of each session.

                                Re-figure as you "age," as you can reclassify your "lifestyle" of
                                activity, or as you have a marked decline in your resting heart rate.

For example: Chris is 20 years old, a moderately active person (70-75% range), with a resting heart rate of 62.

A. 220 – 20 = 200 MHR

B. 200 – 62 = 138 Heart Rate Reserve

C. 138 × .70 = 96 + 62 = 158*
   138 × .75 = 104 + 62 = 166*) Target Heart Rate Training Zone

If Chris keeps working (aerobically exercising) at the range of 158 to 166 heartbeats per minute, the heart would be safely working toward the training effect.

Taking a Count After an Aerobics Interval

As you are beginning an aerobics program, you will want to monitor your pace several times during the workout hour so you can learn constant endurance pacing. Mentally remember your readings, and record them at the end of class.

When you take a pulse rate during the learning process and find that your pace is *below* your established training zone, increase your intensity. If you have a pulse rate *higher* than your established training zone, lower your intensity.

To become familiar with your own response to various intensity levels so you can better regulate yourself, ask yourself, "How do I feel when I get this pulse?" Focus not only on your pulse count but also on what feelings and conditions the number relates to, so you can begin to recognize the signals your body sends. This will also help prepare you to use the RPE monitoring method of intensity, which, as you become a more advanced exerciser, will be a more practical and practiced method than counting your heart rate beats per minute.

Continuing at a pace that is too intense will prove to be an *anaerobic* exercise program. *Anaerobic* activity is basically stop and start, in which the heart is not kept at a constant, steady pace for 20 to 60 minutes. Thus, anaerobic describes an activity that requires all-out effort of short duration and does not utilize oxygen to produce energy. This type of exercise quickly uses up more oxygen than the body can take in while engaging in the exercise, causing an oxygen debt. This, in turn, causes lactic acids (waste products) to accumulate in the muscles, which leads to exhaustion.

The pulse-monitoring procedure during aerobics is then to slow down, walk around, find your pulse, and count it for either 6 or 10 seconds. Each of these counts has been found to be a scientifically accurate measurement for aerobic activity pulse rates. Taking a timed count of greater than 10 seconds immediately after aerobic exercise will tend to be inaccurate

because the heart rate slows down to a *recovery* pulse rather rapidly. You or your instructor will determine whether you will count for 6 or 10 seconds. Immediately following the aerobic exercise segment, count your pulse and multiply the number you get times 10 if using the 6-second count, or times 6 if using a 10-second count. Each of these newly multiplied numbers will equal heartbeats per minute and hopefully will always be in your training zone.

NOTE: *Taking a 6-second count is easy. All you do is add a zero to the pulse you feel, and record that number. You must carefully begin and end exactly with a timer.*

Table 2.1 lists target heart rate counts for individuals who wish to attain fitness using the ideal aerobic range for most people (60–75% of heart rate reserve). Locate the column across the top that is closest to your age and the row down the left side reflecting a figure closest to your resting heart rate. The box where the column and row intersect is *your 10-second target heart rate training zone.*

As your cardiorespiratory system becomes more fit and efficient, work (exercise) will become easier, and you will have to increase the intensity of your activities. Techniques for increasing and decreasing the intensity of your workout will be explained in Chapter 4. By using the target heart rate training zone, you automatically compensate for increased fitness and still maintain the same training effect. Thus, your heart rate will increase during vigorous aerobic activity and should return to normal (pre-activity heart rate) within a short time after the workout. As a rule, the faster it slows down (recovers from exercise), the more physically fit you are, for recovery heart rate improvement is another indication of increased fitness level.

TABLE 2.1   Target Heart Rate Training Zones*

*The numbers in the squares represent pulse beats counted in ten seconds.

Your Age

		15	20	25	30	35	40	45	50	55	60	65	70	75	80
Your average Resting Heart Rate per minute	90	27-29	26-29	26-28	25-28	25-27	24-26	23-26	23-25	22-24	22-24	21-23	21-22	20-22	20-21
	85	26-29	26-29	25-28	25-27	24-27	24-26	23-25	23-25	22-24	22-24	21-23	21-22	20-22	20-21
	80	26-29	25-28	25-28	24-27	24-26	23-26	23-25	22-25	22-24	21-23	21-23	20-22	20-21	19-21
	75	26-29	25-28	25-28	24-27	24-26	23-26	23-25	22-25	21-24	21-23	20-23	20-22	19-21	19-21
	70	25-29	25-28	24-27	24-27	23-26	23-25	22-25	22-24	21-24	21-24	20-22	20-22	19-21	19-20
	65	25-28	25-28	24-27	23-26	23-26	22-25	21-24	21-24	21-23	20-23	20-22	19-21	19-21	18-20
	60	25-28	24-28	24-27	23-26	23-26	22-25	21-24	21-24	20-23	20-22	19-22	19-21	18-21	18-20
	55	24-27	23-27	23-27	23-26	22-25	21-24	21-24	21-24	20-23	20-22	19-22	19-21	18-20	18-20
	50	24-28	23-27	23-26	22-26	22-25	21-25	21-24	20-23	20-23	19-22	19-21	18-21	18-20	17-20

The Borg Scale: Ratings of Perceived Exertion

The second method for monitoring intensity utilizes the psychophysical Borg scale for ratings of perceived exertion (RPE),[19] as shown in Figure 2.4. This scale is based on the finding that, while exercising, one has the ability to accurately assess how hard the body is working. It is basically a judgment call and is more appropriate when used by individuals who have been exercising for a while. The untrained exerciser typically reports a higher RPE than an athlete at the same exercise heart rate.

RPE seems to correlate strongly with other workload indicators, such as ventilation, oxygen consumption, and muscle metabolism. Participants tune into the overall sensation of effort exerted by their entire body, rather than one factor such as local calf or hamstring exhaustion, panting, sweating, or body temperature. When used along with heart rate monitoring, RPE is useful for the novice, who may not yet be aware of how exercise is supposed to feel.

You might begin to make mental notes to yourself during the workout hour concerning your ratings of perceived exertion. After the workout, immediately record what you felt for each phase of the workout, expressed as numbers from 0 to 10. Begin to notice the correlation between target heart rates achieved and how ratings of perceived exertion feel.

The Talk Test

A third and less formal method for determining aerobic intensity is called the *talk test*. It is based on the premise that, while exercising, the participant should always be able to hold a conversation. If the participant can gasp out only one or two words at a time, the exercise intensity is probably anaerobic and should be adjusted to allow for two- to three-word phrases. Because the accuracy of the talk test varies within any given population, it is best utilized in conjunction with the THR and the RPE for monitoring exercise intensity.[20]

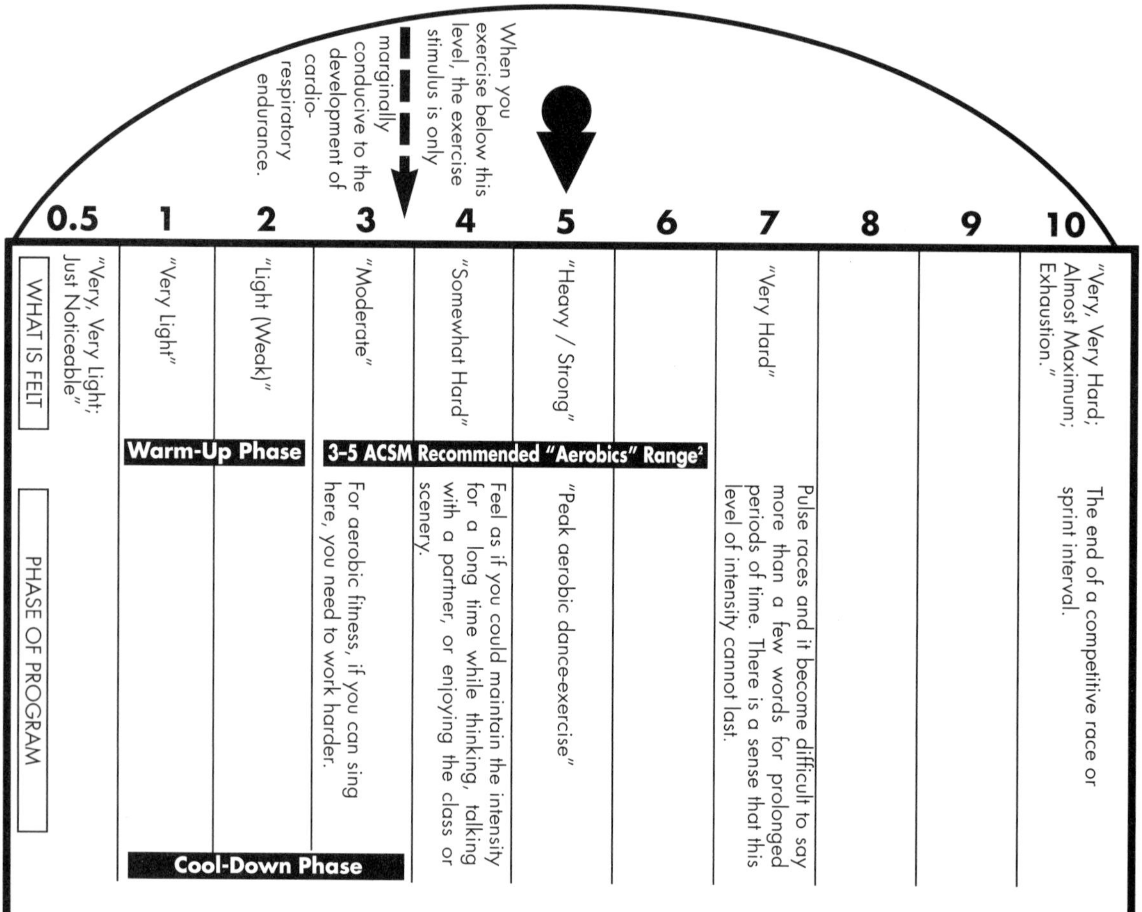

WHAT IS FELT	PHASE OF PROGRAM	0.5	1	2	3	4	5	6	7	8	9	10

When you exercise below this level, the exercise stimulus is only marginally conducive to the development of cardio-respiratory endurance.

"Very, Very Light; Just Noticeable"

"Very Light"

"Light (Weak)"

"Moderate"

"Somewhat Hard"

"Heavy / Strong"

"Very Hard"

"Very, Very Hard; Almost Maximum; Exhaustion."

Warm-Up Phase

3-5 ACSM Recommended "Aerobics" Range[2]

For aerobic fitness, if you can sing here, you need to work harder.

Feel as if you could maintain the intensity for a long time while thinking, talking with a partner, or enjoying the class or scenery.

"Peak aerobic dance-exercise"

Pulse races and it become difficult to say more than a few words for prolonged periods of time. There is a sense that this level of intensity cannot last.

The end of a competitive race or sprint interval.

Cool-Down Phase

Figure 2.4. Borg Scale ratings of perceived exertion

Which Method Is Best?

The experts do not agree when it comes to THR versus RPE. Some claim that only THR methods are accurate; others believe that RPE and the talk test are more practical. Because all the methods are useful and none is consistently ideal, a good solution is to *use a combination of all three*. Once a participant has developed a good understanding of the heart rate/RPE relationship, heart rate can be monitored less frequently and RPE can be used as a primary means of measuring exercise intensity with the talk test as an informal supplemental backup measure.[21]

IMPACT: HIGH, LOW, COMBINATION HIGH/LOW, AND MODERATE

There is one more ingredient in the aerobics formula for fitness to consider when establishing your prescription for exercise of how often (frequency), how much work (heart rate beats per minute/intensity), and how long to work out (duration of time per session). This ingredient is the concept of *impact* and needs to be included when determining the time duration you spend per session of aerobic exercise.

Basic step movements in aerobics have changed considerably since the origin of the activity. These changes have centered on injury reduction and prevention, with primary focus on the amount of vertical force exerted on the feet as they contact (impact) with the floor surface and how this stress subsequently effects the musculoskeletal system.

Early programs included many steps and gestures with great bodily elevation and with a corresponding great compression upon foot contact with the floor. Research has given the aerobics enthusiast a variety of safe alternatives regarding impact and movement possibilities.

IMPACT EVALUATION

High-Impact Aerobics (HIA)

High-impact aerobics (HIA) involves steps and gestures in which both feet may be off the floor at the same time briefly. This step and gesture movement selection results in great force exerted when the foot meets the floor surface. This force is absorbed by the landing, floor surface, shoes, orthotics (if worn), and musculoskeletal system (muscles, tendons, ligaments, joints, and bones).

Several examples of basic movements that are considered high-impact are jogging, hopping, and jumping. A few characteristics of high-impact aerobics are:

- Music between 130 and 160 beats per minute (bpm).
- Faster music, smaller moves.
- Slower music, greater range of motion.
- Land through toe/ball/heel.
- Avoid over 8 repetitions (reps) on one limb.
- Strengthen anterior tibialis (shin area).
- Strengthen hamstrings.
- Limit to every other day.
- Higher intensity = $>VO_2$ max.

- Moderate intensity = > fat utilization.[22]

High-impact aerobics is generally *not recommended* for:

- Individuals who are obviously deconditioned or out of shape, especially those who are obese.
- Anyone who is susceptible to specific injuries (such as shin splints) caused by, or likely to be aggravated by, upward impacts on the feet.
- Women in the latter stages of pregnancy, who usually have loosening of the joints.
- Individuals who are incontinent.
- Participants who are uncomfortable with high-impact steps.[23]

Low-Impact Aerobics (LIA)

Low-impact aerobics (LIA) involves steps and gestures that produce less force when the foot strikes the floor than those in high-impact movements. Great control over the landing and force of foot impact is present, because one foot is in contact with the floor at all times.

Low-impact does not mean low-intensity! Cardiorespiratory conditioning can still be achieved as long as you are working within the target heart rate training zone you've established. To help elevate your heart rate if it is not in your zone, place more emphasis on weight-bearing moves that lower your center of gravity. Deepening knee flexion (bending motions) that use the large leg and buttocks muscles (quadriceps and hamstrings, and gluteals) and gesture actions of the upper body are ways to accomplish this. Examples of low-impact moves are step-touch, lunge, grapevine, marching, and vigorous walking in place. Characteristics of low-impact aerobics are:

- Heart rate is kept in the target heart rate training zone.
- Moves can be modified if THR is not maintained.
- Any tempo music can be utilized.

- For faster tempos, cover less space.

- For slower tempos, cover more space.

- Keep feet closer to the ground to decrease impact.

- Use moves traveling from side-to-side and forward-and-back so large muscles of legs and trunk are engaged continuously.

- Make controlled, vigorous arm movements to compensate for the reduction in activity of the leg and back muscles when the height of hops and jumps is reduced. "Research has shown that up to 25% more work can be performed with the arms and legs combined, compared to work performed by the legs alone.[24]

- Avoid using the arms above shoulder level for extended periods. "Doing so necessitates extended isometric contractions of the arm and shoulder muscles and probably causes greater after-exercise soreness. In addition, holding the arms over the head raises blood pressure, and anyone with high blood pressure or a history of angina pectoralis should be discouraged from doing these movements.[25]

- Turn toes/knees out with wide legs.

- Raise and lower the center of gravity.

- In lateral moves, keep legs turned out.

- Make angle of knee flexion 90 degrees.

- Strengthen both vastus medialis (front, inner thigh) and hamstrings.

- Use adductor muscles for correct mechanics.[26]

Low-impact aerobics (LIA) is generally *not recommended* for:

- Anyone who complains of knee discomfort during prolonged knee flexion.

- Individuals who have severely flattened or pronated feet. (Knee flexion, and some side-to-side movements in which one foot crosses in front of the other, tend to produce a shifting of the kneecap toward the outer side of the knee joint, which increases stress.)

- Well-conditioned, injury-free individuals who are unable to achieve their target heart rate, even in the most intense LIA program. (Although many instructors use LIA exclusively in the interest of safety, conventional high-impact choreography may be acceptable for these participants as long as they remain injury-free.[27])

Combination High-/Low-Impact Aerobics (CIA or Combo-Impact)

The combination style of choreography utilizes characteristics of both high- and low-impact movement and can be a safe and exciting blend. Combination high/low impact choreography can be defined in two ways:[28]

1. *Routines that offer both a high-impact and a low-impact version of a movement.* Programs that offer both of these work best in classes with mixed fitness levels so individual participants can select the amount of impact appropriate for them. A beginner in such a program, therefore, may choose to perform the low-impact version whereas an experienced dance-exerciser may feel more challenged by the high-impact movements.

2. *Routines combining a series of varied high-impact and a series of varied low-impact movements.* This style lends itself well to classes of experienced aerobic dance-exercisers whose primary concern is to improve cardiorespiratory fitness while minimizing the risk of injury.

Combo-impact aerobics offers a wide range of choices and possibilities. It allows you to individualize how much physical stress you choose to safely experience at various times and stages of your life according to your fitness level, personal goals, and special interests. Especially if you are a beginner, coming off an illness or injury, obese, older, or a pregnant woman, you will want to choose the less biomechanically stressful low-impact movements. Athletes in training and well-conditioned injury-free individuals may choose the high-impact movements and series more frequently, or even exclusively. As another option, they may wish to blend their HIA and LIA techniques into the *moderate-impact aerobic* (MIA) style explained in the next section.

The unique feature of a combination approach is that participants can choose from the various possibilities the impact that best fits their current lifestyle needs. Some people, of course, can never participate in the high-impact movements, because of permanent physical limitations.

A three-step process for interpreting high-impact steps into an acceptable low-impact movement (Figures 2.5–2.8) will be accomplished by:

■ Lowering the foot impact.

■ Increasing the arm movement.

■ Increasing the use of space.

Step 1 of this process minimizes the impact, and steps 2 and 3 increase the intensity of the movement. The idea is to change one element at a time. First, lower the foot impact by keeping the feet closer to the floor. Second, exaggerate the original arm movement. Finally, increase the use of space by covering more ground with each

step. Keen attention to the beat of the music becomes important when converting high-impact movement to low, to ensure an injury-free workout.

Combining a series of varied high-impact and a series of varied low-impact movements will produce fewer of the large upward impacts typical of an HIA program and fewer of the large side-to-side impacts typical of many LIA programs. A key to remember is that it is the sum total of all the stresses on the various vulnerable parts of the body that determines whether injury occurs.

Moderate-Impact Aerobics (MIA)

The fourth and the newest alternative style of impact aerobics is called moderate-impact aerobics (MIA). It was designed as the result of laboratory and dance-exercise class research done at San Diego State University.[29] By adapting the gesture style (non-weight-bearing body parts) and foot impact, this choreographic style combines the best elements of both HIA and LIA, for movements that keep the intensity needed to maintain target heart rate while reducing foot-impact forces.

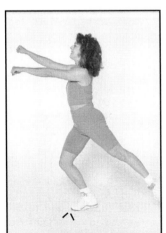 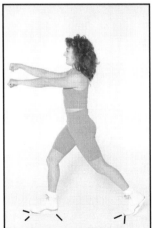 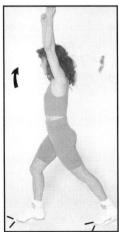 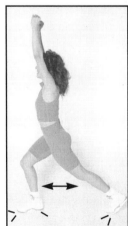

Figure 2.5. High-impact version of the lunge. The exerciser jumps high in the air when moving from side to side.

Figure 2.6. Impact is lowered by stepping outward instead of jumping.

Figure 2.7. Intensity is increased by raising the arms above the shoulders.

Figure 2.8. Increased use of space occurs by reaching out farther every step.

The key technique to master is called *plyo-metric*.[30] At least one foot remains in contact with the floor most of the time in order to reduce potentially injurious stresses on the body. However, the center of gravity of the body rises and falls almost as much as it does during HIA, thus avoiding prolonged knee flexion.[31] This raising and lowering of the center of gravity, by extending the hip, knee, and ankle joints without actually leaving the floor, requires *work*, the expenditure of energy. This will provide for a relatively high exercise intensity.

Plyometric technique has been used for many years by athletes, in such sports as track and skiing, to increase power in a workout. These athletes have used plyometric techniques to increase their springing or bounding abilities. For example, picture yourself engaged in either sport and landing and recovering after a forceful jump move. When you lift and spring off the ground, that action is called plyometric. You are in fact forcefully loading the weight as you jump and then have a powerful unloading, or springing out of this move.[32]

Although this is a very effective method to increase power, it can be very stressful to the musculoskeletal system of the average person. So in moderate-impact aerobics this plyometric principle of power in movement will be used, but you will load the weight with much less force by simply bending or flexing the knees and the hips, and then springing out of this position.

This allows you to safely increase the intensity, and also safely increase power in your leg and hip muscles.

In many LIA routines, the emphasis is placed on flexing the knees so that the body is lowered and then raised to an erect position. This can be stressful to the knees of some participants. In addition, many beginners have found that this *down-up* movement is rather unnatural and requires a great deal of concentration. If the amount of knee flexion is decreased and *emphasis is placed on extending the knees and ankle joints without the feet actually leaving the floor* — as in moderate-impact aerobics — the center of

gravity can be raised and lowered effectively. The physiological cost is quite high, but the bouncy motions are comfortable and stimulating for many participants.[33]

To clarify the differences between the three distinct methods of impact, here's an example of *stepping-in-place*:

- **High-impact aerobics:** jogging — both feet off the ground briefly.

- **Low-impact aerobics:** marching — one foot always in contact with the floor.

- **Moderate-impact aerobics:** plyometric techniques using the lift and spring action (see Figure 2.9).

The main difference between high-impact jogging and the moderate-impact version is the *rate at which the force is increased on the foot*. Even though the final load on the foot for the MIA step is close in magnitude to that for the HIA step, the load increased much more gradually during the MIA step.

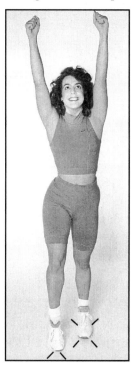

Figure 2.9. Keeping your right foot flat on the floor, raise your left foot until the tip of your left toe is just barely in contact with the floor. Now alternate the position of the feet to the same tempo that you used for the two previous movements. Lift your body as high as possible as you shift your weight from foot to foot by using the full range of motion of your ankle joints and moderate amounts of knee flexion and extension. Make certain that the heel of the supporting foot is pressed to the floor to maintain a good range of motion of the ankle joint.

Researchers believe that when high levels of force are exerted on the feet suddenly, the human body is vulnerable to injury. The body is equipped with reflex mechanisms that can control muscle contractions to protect it from mechanical stress. Damage can occur, however, if the forces reach high levels before the reflex mechanisms can provide protection. In practical terms, the springlike motions of MIA are less jarring than the high-impact versions because the body is raised and lowered with control. In HIA, the body is under less control as it falls freely, colliding suddenly with the floor.[34]

Guidelines For Using Moderate-Impact Aerobics

1. Begin movements by lifting your body upward, rising onto the balls of your feet. Complete each step, whenever possible, by lowering your heels and gently pressing them against the floor. This pressing action produces the spring-like motion characteristic of MIA steps. The lifting and lowering of the center of gravity is what increases exercise intensity.

2. Concentrate on leaving at least one foot on the floor most of the time. The purpose of MIA is to reduce the magnitude of impact. Steps such as MIA jogs, jumps, and twists are performed with both feet on the floor, either bearing the weight on both feet, as in a jump, or bearing it on one foot with the second foot lightly touching the floor, as in a twisting step.

   MIA steps that require lifting one foot off the floor, such as kicks and knee-lifts, must be carefully timed so the airborne foot is back on the floor before the opposite foot leaves the floor.

3. Exercise intensity can be increased by directionally traveling across the floor and using the arms through a wide range of movement.

4. To adapt your present LIA or HIA moves to MIA, concentrate on taking the movement up and down while keeping one foot on the floor most of the time. (Not all LIA and HIA steps can be modified to suit MIA. Practice and common sense will help you determine which steps adjust best.) Examples of steps that adapt well to MIA are heel-jacks, jogs, jumps, kicks, knee-lifts, ponies, step-touches, and twists.

5. For variety, mix MIA with LIA and HIA steps.

6. Because the ankle joint is used through a wider range of motion with MIA than with HIA and LIA, it is particularly important to strengthen the tibialis anterior (shin area) and stretch the gastrocnemius and soleus (posterior, lower leg area) muscles during warm-up and cool-down. These precautions will help prevent tightness of the calf and muscle imbalance.[35]

CALORIC EXPENDITURE FROM AEROBICS

Recent research has indicated that, if all of the variables are carefully attended to and duplicated, aerobics can cause substantial energy expenditure of more than 12 calories per minute, with no significant difference in caloric expenditure between low- and high-impact routines (if these routines are duplicated in style, content, and energy level).[36] This study was carried out using certified instructors (IDEA Foundation and/or AFAA) and involved two 11-minute sequences of high-impact and low-impact aerobic dance-exercise, at a tempo of 148 bpm. For those concerned with weight management, it is exciting to conclude that one can engage in high- or low-impact moves and still significantly expend energy and burn calories.

Because the average peak force of LIA can result in impact forces of approximately 1½ times your weight and HIA can result in foot impact approximately 3 times your weight,[37] the impact you choose can be important — especially if you have physical limitations (e.g., obesity, pregnancy, susceptibility to joint injury). Choice of impact, therefore, does not have to be made in regard to caloric expenditure.

TOTAL PHYSICAL FITNESS: A CHOICE

Achieving physical fitness requires dedication to personal excellence. There are few shortcuts but many pleasurable alternatives. Once achieved, you must continue to make choices that maintain your fitness for a lifetime. Fitness is a journey — a continual process — not just one achieved destination. Maintaining fitness is a lot easier than initially achieving it, though you also will discover that the less physically fit you are, the longer it will take you to become fit.

The total physical fitness journey requires:

- seeking valid information;
- establishing your starting points;
- setting reasonable and challenging goals;
- monitoring your daily progress;
- continually making self-disciplined choices from the imaged pictures you make in your head and your self-talk, to the motivated aerobic exercise moves you make.

Enjoy the journey!

■ ■ ■

You alone are the Captain of your ship.
You alone control the choices.
No one, and nothing else
can do it for you . . .

■ ■ ■

Finding the courage to change,
is no more difficult than
learning to make one
small choice at a time.

■ ■ ■

One simple decision:
  consciously
    actively
      make your choices.

Choices, Shad Helmstetter

■ ■ ■

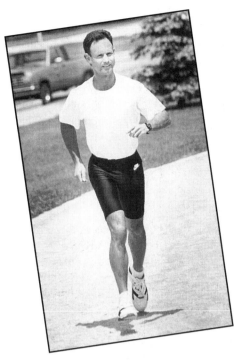

3

Fitness Testing Determines Your Starting Point

The next step in the journey toward achieving and then maintaining physical fitness for a lifetime involves establishing your current fitness starting point, using scientific test and assessment procedures. Clearly knowing yourself in terms of your past history, risk factors, and present physical status will assist you in developing a lifetime fitness plan. It will enable you to not only realistically and safely set achievable short-term fitness goals but also will provide the basis for continually motivating you to adhere to the program you do establish to achieve your long-range and lifetime fitness goals.

You initially may find that it can be painful and devastating to realize that you are out of shape and test poorly on a laboratory or field stress test. No one really wants to see or hear or feel scientific results that label them inferior or below the norm. But having the determination and courage to find out just where you are at the outset and then, with time and dedication, progressing to the point where your post-assessment test numbers represent an excellent state of fitness and well-being is motivating and is the ink needed to permanently blueprint your desired changes for a lifetime.

In most instances, specific fitness testing is appropriate only after obtaining a medical history. Screening may uncover any potential problems and determine if you should be considered for a specific exercise prescription. Most course settings require this pre-screening, or a thorough medical exam, if you have any limitations or known risk factors.

UNDERSTANDING FITNESS ASSESSMENTS

The purpose of an initial pre-course fitness assessment is to establish a baseline of information from which later changes can be compared. Assessment principles include the following:

1. Nearly all assessment protocols result in *estimated* values for the fitness component being measured. So consider the testing as merely an effective way to measure your improvement in your performance over time, and not as an absolutely correct physiologic measurement or comparison.

2. By following consistent procedures of testing (using the same test, person administering it,

instrument, time of day, etc.), you are more assured of accuracy in measurement over time.

3. Results are recorded for comparison purposes. The person being tested should understand these values and ask questions as needed to ensure understanding.

MEASURING AEROBIC CAPACITY

Pre-assessing your current status by having a thorough physical fitness exam will measure your heart's response to increasing amounts of exercise (work, stress) by measuring your ability to use oxygen. Physical fitness can and should be measured in one of two ways at least every three years:

■ A laboratory physical fitness test.

■ A field test administered by you and a friend.

The Laboratory Physical Fitness Test

The "master key" to good health and exercising without fear is a properly conducted treadmill stress test to check out the precise condition of your heart.[1] Physical fitness and health are different, and the treadmill stress ECG helps to make that distinction.[2]

Prior to a treadmill stress test, you will be thoroughly screened. This consists of: (a) a brief history-taking and physical exam during which the technician listens to your heart and lungs; (b) a check for the use of drugs known to affect the ECG (e.g., various heart and hypertensive medications); (c) a check for history of congenital or acquired heart disorders; and (d) an evaluation of the resting ECG.

This screening and background check will help to determine your risk factors. A risk factor is a feature in a person's heredity, background, or present lifestyle that increases the likelihood of developing coronary heart disease. If no risk factors are present, an exercise test usually is not necessary below age thirty-five if guidelines mentioned in Chapter 2 are followed. If symptoms of heart, lung, or metabolic disease are present, a maximum stress test is recommended for individuals of any age prior to the onset of a vigorous exercise program, and followed with tests every two years.[3]

Sub-Maximal Testing

Sub-maximal testing is accomplished by means of a physical fitness test (stress test) on a treadmill. Electrocardiogram leads transmit and record electrical (heart) impulses that are read on a machine and recorded on a strip of paper. You are tested only to approximately 150 beats per minute, not to exhaustion.

The ECG electrodes with leads are circular rubber discs with wires attached to them. The discs are glued onto the chest and back at key locations so various "pictures" of your heart, from different angles and sides, can all be recorded at once. Usually between seven and ten electrodes are applied, depending on the laboratory's procedures or on the individual's specific needs.

You probably will be asked to walk at a pace of 3.3 miles per hour (90 meters per minute) on the treadmill. The grade will begin flat and will increase slowly in gradation, as if you were walking up a hill. Every minute the "hill" will become steeper and more difficult to climb. When your heart rate reaches 150 beats per minute, a record is made of the amount of time it took for you to arrive at that reading. Then, through an indirect method of extrapolation (projection of maximum results through having tested many others the same way in the past), your fitness ability is estimated.

Basically, the longer it takes your heart rate to reach 150 beats per minute, the more fit you are; the shorter it takes, the less fit you are. Sub-maximal fitness testing usually is used with those who know of no outstanding limitations and who are interested in starting an aerobics program.

Maximal Testing

Maximal testing procedures are administered if an individual's need is more specific (i.e., for diagnostic or research purposes). Maximum testing directly reveals how much oxygen you use, because you are tested to exhaustion. The "exhaustion" point is when you start to get markedly fatigued. Some researchers believe that maximum laboratory testing is the *only* conclusive type to use.

Field Tests of Fitness

You may not have immediate access to a laboratory and qualified physiologists to monitor the results recorded with the treadmill method. Therefore, field tests have been developed to help you assess your own physical fitness by determining your current aerobic capacity. This testing is easily conducted in an aerobics class setting.

The following information and Tables 3.1 and 3.2 were developed from Dr. Kenneth Cooper's book, *The Aerobics Program for Total Well-Being*.[4] Cooper's 12-Minute Test and 1.5-Mile Test are two that you can administer by yourself or with the help of a friend. You should assess your cardiorespiratory endurance using one of these tests before you begin your aerobics program and reassess your cardiorespiratory efficiency eight weeks later. As aerobics becomes a lifetime activity for you, an ongoing assessment should be done every two months, and your results compared with those from your first assessment. This also will help you set continual, lifelong, specific physical fitness goals.

As guidelines for field-testing:

1. If you previously have been physically inactive, participate in one to two weeks of walking or slow jogging before undertaking either of Cooper's tests.

2. Wear loose clothing in which you can freely sweat, and a sport shoe that conforms to the guidelines suggested in Chapter 6.

NOTE: If you are over age thirty-five, you should start an aerobics program by first seeing your doctor and then taking a monitored laboratory fitness test. Individuals with known cardiovascular, pulmonary, or metabolic disease should have a maximum stress test prior to beginning vigorous exercise at any age. These people and those whose exercise tests are abnormal should get a stress test annually.

3. Determine first which field test you plan to take. You can choose running with time or distance as the stopping point.
   - If time is the stopping point, take the 12-minute test.
   - If distance is the stopping point, take the 1.5-mile test.
   - If you believe rather strongly that you are really out of shape, the 12-minute test will be easier because you run for this amount of time only. (An individual might take 20 minutes to complete 1.5 miles.)

4. Be sure that you have a stopwatch or a second-hand on your watch, or that you are close to a wall timer.

5. Immediately before performing the test, spend five to ten minutes warming up the muscles (see Chapter 7).

6. Have a partner record your data (as time it takes or laps or distance).

7. Run or walk (or a combination) as quickly as you can for 12 minutes or 1.5 miles. (See Figure 3.1.) This is an all-out test of endurance.

8. When you stop, identify precisely the distance covered in miles and tenths of miles or time it took, and have your partner record it.

9. Be sure to cool down by first walking slowly for several minutes, and then finish by doing cool-down stretching.

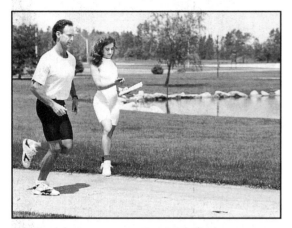

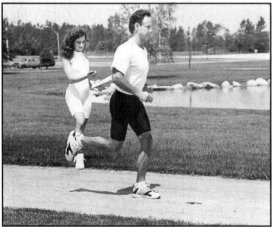

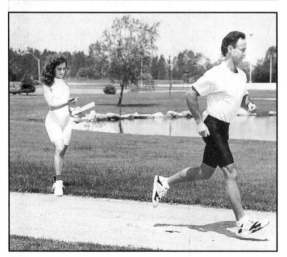

Figure 3.1. Field testing to determine your aerobic fitness starting point.

10. Interpret your results for the specific test you used, in the forms provided at the end of the chapter. At the conclusion of your course, reassess your fitness. What change did you experience from the Pre-Test to Post-Test?

For some beginners, the "good" performance level is high. Do not be discouraged. You will be pleased with your improvement as you participate in a regular aerobics program.

FITNESS FOR LIFE

Attaining a level of physical fitness labeled "good" or "high" (lab tests), or "good," "excellent," or "superior" (field tests) does not mean you have achieved a finished product or goal. Instead, you have found a method of getting in shape that must be continued for the rest of your life. If you discontinue your program completely, all your aerobic gains will be lost in ten weeks.[5]

The need for personal fitness must result in a complete change in lifestyle. You must prioritize and program exercise into your busy weekly schedule for the rest of your life. A "yo-yo" concept of a 10-week class now, and maybe one a year later, just doesn't maintain fitness and a healthy heart.

SUMMARY

You have just completed assessing your aerobic capacity. With this information, you can establish your cardiovascular fitness goal. Setting goals helps to keep you focused on daily improvement and positive change. It encourages consistency in your fitness program and helps to keep you on target because without goals there's nothing to shoot for!

Write one fitness goal to be achieved by the end of this course. Truly stretch yourself and your potential in regard to what you are actually capable of achieving.

TABLE 3.1   Cooper's 12-Minute Walking/Running Test[6]

Fitness Category		Age (years)					
		13-19	**20-29**	**30-39**	**40-49**	**50-59**	**60 +**
		Distance (Miles) Covered in 12 Minutes					
I. Very Poor	(men)	<1.30	<1.22	<1.18	<1.14	<1.03	< .87
	(women)	<1.0	< .96	< .94	< .88	< .84	< .78
II. Poor	(men)	1.30-1.37	1.22-1.31	1.18-1.30	1.14-1.24	1.03-1.16	.87-1.02
	(women)	1.00-1.18	.96-1.11	.95-1.05	.88- .98	.84- .93	.78- .86
III. Fair	(men)	1.38-1.56	1.32-1.49	1.31-1.45	1.25-1.39	1.17-1.30	1.03-1.20
	(women)	1.19-1.29	1.12-1.22	1.06-1.18	.99-1.11	.94-1.05	.87- .98
IV. Good	(men)	1.57-1.72	1.50-1.64	1.46-1.56	1.40-1.53	1.31-1.44	1.21-1.32
	(women)	1.30-1.43	1.23-1.34	1.19-1.29	1.12-1.24	1.06-1.18	.99-1.09
V. Excellent	(men)	1.73-1.86	1.65-1.76	1.57-1.69	1.54-1.65	1.45-1.58	1.33-1.55
	(women)	1.44-1.51	1.35-1.45	1.30-1.39	1.25-1.34	1.19-1.30	1.10-1.18
VI. Superior	(men)	>1.87	>1.77	>1.70	>1.66	>1.59	>1.56
	(women)	>1.52	>1.46	>1.40	>1.35	>1.31	>1.19

< = less than;   > = more than.

From *The Aerobics Program For Total Well-Being*, by Kenneth H. Cooper, M.D., M.P.H. Copyright 1982 by Kenneth H. Cooper. Reprinted by permission of the publisher, Bantam-Doubleday-Dell, New York, NY 10103.

PRE-TEST

Start Time: _____   Stop Time: _____   Distance Covered: _____

Circle Fitness Category: Very Poor   Poor   Fair   Good   Excellent   Superior

GOAL: _____

POST-TEST

Start Time: _____   Stop Time: _____   Distance Covered: _____

Circle Fitness Category: Very Poor   Poor   Fair   Good   Excellent   Superior

GOAL: _____

TABLE 3.2　　Cooper's 1.5-Mile Run/Walk Test

Fitness Category		Age (years)					
		13-19	20-29	30-39	40-49	50-59	60 +
		Time (Minutes)[7]					
I. Very Poor	(men)	>15:31	>16:01	>16:31	>17:31	>19:01	>20:01
	(women)	>18:31	>19:01	>19:31	>20:01	>20:31	>21:01
II. Poor	(men)	12:11-15:30	14:01-16:00	14:44-16:30	15:36-17:30	17:01-19:00	19:01-20:00
	(women)	16:55-18:30	18:31-19:00	19:01-19:30	19:31-20:00	20:01-20:30	21:00-21:31
III. Fair	(men)	10:49-12:10	12:01-14:00	12:31-14:45	13:01-15:35	14:31-17:00	16:16-19:00
	(women)	14:31-16:54	15:55-18:30	16:31-19:00	17:31-19:30	19:01-20:00	19:31-20:30
IV. Good	(men)	9:41-10:48	10:46-12:00	11:01-12:30	11:31-13:00	12:31-14:30	14:00-16:15
	(women)	12:30-14:30	13:31-15:54	14:31-16:30	15:56-17:30	16:31-19:00	17:31-19:30
V. Excellent	(men)	8:37- 9:40	9:45-10:45	10:00-11:00	10:30-11:30	11:00-12:30	11:15-13:59
	(women)	11:50-12:29	12:30-13:30	13:00-14:30	13:45-15:55	14:30-16:30	16:30-17:30
VI. Superior	(men)	< 8:37	< 9:45	<10:00	<10:30	<11:00	<11:15
	(women)	<11:50	<12:30	<13:00	<13:45	<14:30	<16:30

< = less than;　> = more than.

From *The Aerobics Program For Total Well-Being*, by Kenneth H. Cooper, M.D., M.P.H. Copyright 1982 by Kenneth H. Cooper. Reprinted by permission of the publisher, Bantam-Doubleday-Dell, New York, NY 10103.

PRE-TEST

Check Off Laps (e.g., 14 for 190-yard track; 21 for 126-yard track):

1 - 2 - 3 - 4 - 5 - 6 - 7 - 8 - 9 - 10 - 11 - 12 - 13 - 14 - 15 - 16 - 17 - 18 - 19 - 20 - 21

Time: _____　OR:

Just record here if using an open roadway.

　　　Stop Time: _____

　　　−Start Time: _____

　　　Time: _____

Circle Fitness Category:

Very Poor　　Poor　　Fair

Good　　Excellent　　Superior

GOAL: _____

POST-TEST

Check Off Laps (e.g., 14 for 190-yard track; 21 for 126-yard track):

1 - 2 - 3 - 4 - 5 - 6 - 7 - 8 - 9 - 10 - 11 - 12 - 13 - 14 - 15 - 16 - 17 - 18 - 19 - 20 - 21

Time: _____　OR:

Just record here if using an open roadway.

　　　Stop Time: _____

　　　−Start Time: _____

　　　Time: _____

Circle Fitness Category:

Very Poor　　Poor　　Fair

Good　　Excellent　　Superior

GOAL: _____

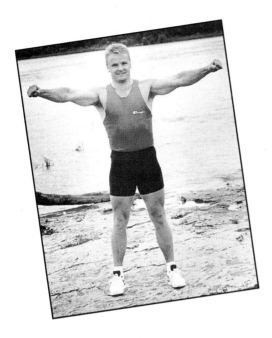

4

Principles of Aerobics Programs

The foundation for understanding physical fitness has been set. Your mind is set, the basic new terminologies have been defined, and you have established your cardiovascular starting point in order to set your goal. It's now time to build upon this foundation that represents a safe, beneficial, and fun total fitness workout session.

AEROBICS PROGRAMMING

Each aerobics class workout session is structured into four basic segments: warm-up; aerobics; strength training; and cool down, flexibility training, and relaxation. Each of these segments is further structured into specific activities. Principles and guidelines are given for each.[1, 2, 3, 4, 5]

1 Warm-Up Segment

The warm-up begins with activities that are active, medium-to-low-level, rhythmic, limbering, standing, range-of-motion type of exercises that raise the body's core temperature slightly, initiate muscular movements, and prepare you for more strenuous moves to come. Examples such as step-touch with low arm-circling, strides

with sweeping punches (shown in the chapter opening photo), and other gentle, sweeping motions of low intensity are good to initiate the warm-up. The time-frame can be approximately 5 minutes.

Following the initial warm-up exercises, slow, sustained, static stretching is performed, because the muscles, tendons, ligaments, and joints are now loose and pliable. Static stretching is done from head to toe (Figures 4.1 and 4.2). It is probably the most popular, easiest, and safest form of stretching. It involves gradually stretching a muscle or muscle group to the point of limitation, then holding that position for approximately 15 seconds. The stretch is repeated to the opposite side. Several repetitions of each stretch are performed. Static stretching is recommended when muscles are warm — after the initial active phase of the warm-up and later after intense physical activity.

Breathing should be continuous. Your entire system, especially your working muscles, constantly need oxygen. Holding your breath and turning red is never an appropriate way to exercise. While performing the warm-up (and cool-down) stretching (or any strengthening exercise), you should exhale when you stretch, by puckering your lips and breathing out, and inhale when

**STRETCHING —
From Head
To Toe**

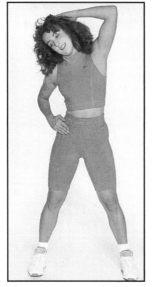

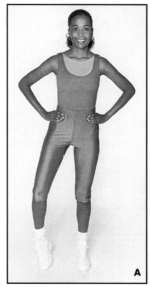

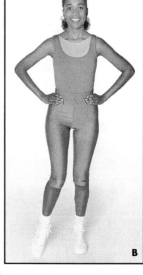

Figure 4.1. Head drop to the side and press.

Figure 4.2. Ankle stretching.

you relax your muscles. Cue yourself: "Breathe out and stretch;" "breathe in and relax."

The time frame suggested for the warm-up stretching segment is approximately 5 minutes.

2 Aerobics Segment

The aerobics segment can be subdivided into six sections, each focusing on the impact in relation to: the heart rate intensity you are building, sustaining, or lowering and according to which phase of the hour you are in. At least two heart-rate checks should be monitored during the segment.

Low-Impact Aerobics Warm-up

These are simple, low-intensity moves that gradually increase your heart rate. They start with the legs down low and arms below heart level. To gradually increase the intensity, the range-of-motion of each movement is first increased, and then the use of air and floor space is widened. For example: Step-touch in place with hand claps, punching, or arms shoulder high

with hands pointing in (Figure 4.3), and then both hands and toe-touch extending far out, to the side. Progress to a grapevine, using large arm reaches (Figure 4.4). The time-frame is approximately 5 minutes.

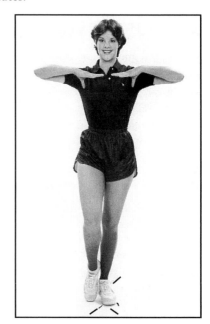

Figure 4.3.
Jazz-Touch-In.

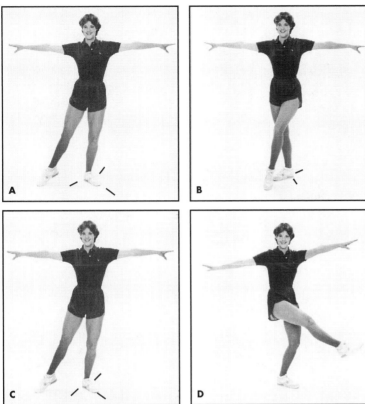

Figure 4.4. The Grapevine (low impact).

Power Low-Impact Aerobics

These moves increase the load on the large muscles of the legs by bending and extending more, with the accent on lifting or raising the center of gravity while keeping at least one foot firmly on the floor and recovering with an ankle-flexion springing movement. Traveling through space is characteristic with these movements, which really challenge the leg muscles. Examples are strong low-impact bouncing and reaching with plyometrics (Figure 4.5), squats or plies (Figure 4.6), lunges, and power walking. The time-frame is approximately 10 minutes.

High/Low-Impact Aerobics

Here you'll intersperse high-impact moves, in which both feet may leave the floor

momentarily, with low-impact moves, in which one foot always remains on the floor. You'll raise your arms overhead more frequently, and raise the knees and feet up higher. A key point in this segment is that the intensity of the moves you choose must remain high so the heart rate maintains the high, but safe, training zone you've established for cardiorespiratory improvement. Not more than four high-impact repetitions are performed on the same leg at one time. The music speed will range between 160 beats per minute, or fewer, for low-impact moves and up to 180 bpm for high-impact exercises. Examples are: two high-impact jacks in the wide-stride-and-together leg and arm positions (Figure 4.7), followed by four power low-impact pace-walking moves with forceful arms (Figure 4.8). The time-frame is approximately 15 minutes.

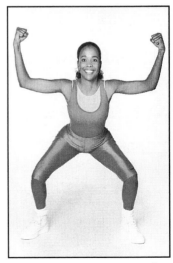

Figure 4.5. Bouncing and reaching (power low impact).

Figure 4.6. Squats (power low impact).

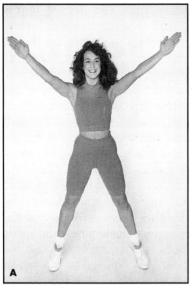

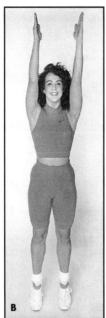

Figure 4.7. Jacks (high/low impact).

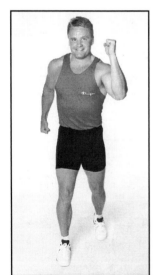

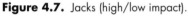

Figure 4.8.
Power pace-walk
(high/low impact).

Power Low-Impact Aerobics

Again, these are the center-of-gravity lifting, hip-knee-ankle extending moves, followed by the knee-flexion, ankle springing-action moves in which one foot is always in contact with the floor, to keep the force of impact low. The time-frame is approximately 5 minutes.

Low-Impact Aerobics Cool-Down

These are the lower intensity moves needed to gradually lower your heart rate. They are still active and rhythmic, using a full range-of-motion, but now are low-level and slower, half-the-tempo moves, such as two-foot bouncing and punching (Figure 4.9), standing upper- and lower-body conditioning moves, such as a squat with bicep curls (Figure 4.10). The time-frame is approximately 10 minutes.

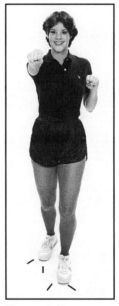

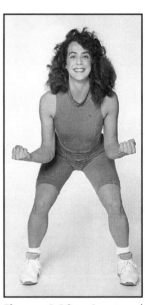

Figure 4.9.
Bouncing (low-impact
cool-down).

Figure 4.10. Squat and
curls (low-impact cool-down).

Post-Aerobic Stretching

Stretching the lower-body muscles to aid blood returning to the heart and preventing blood pooling in the legs is performed by standing static stretches for the hamstrings (Figure 4.11), quadriceps and iliopsoas (Figure 4.12), and calf muscles (Figure 4.13). The time-frame can be approximately 3–5 minutes.

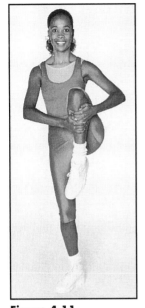

Figure 4.11.
Hamstrings.

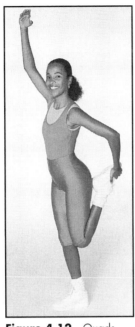

Figure 4.12. Quads.

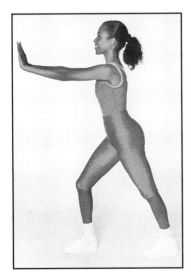

Figure 4.13.
Calves.

included within an aerobics hour focuses on the strength development of isolated muscle groups. It is performed at the end of the aerobics workout but before the final cool-down, flexibility training, and relaxation segment.

The reasoning for this is simple. With an increase in the resistance (weight) that must be applied to any movement for significant change (training) to occur, the workload placed on the heart, lungs, and vascular system also increases. An individual is more readily placed in a breathless "oxygen-debt" state. During the aerobic phase, your goal is *not* to be in a breathless state. You want to be continually working in a breathe-easy state, steadily pacing your intensity.

Sample strength activities for the chest are push-ups (Figure 4.14), for the arms and shoulders, short-lever bicep curls (Figure 4.15) and long-lever lateral raises (Figure 4.16), curl-up

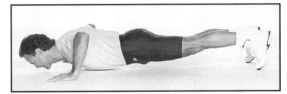

Figure 4.14. Chest — Push-ups.

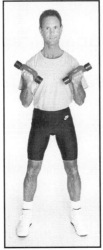

Figure 4.15.
Arms and Shoulders
— Short-lever bicep
curl.

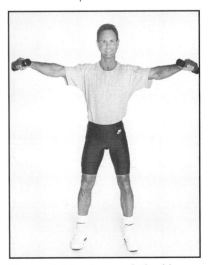

Figure 4.16. Arms and Shoulders —
Long-lever lateral raise.

3   Strength Training and Calisthenics Segment

Although a general strengthening of all the muscles of the body occurs during vigorous aerobics, the optional strength program

variations for the abdomen (Figure 4.17), squats for the buttocks (Figure 4.18), leg curls for the thighs (Figure 4.19), alternating ankle flexion and extension for the shins (Figure 4.20), and one-legged calf raises for the calves (Figure 4.21).

These all represent isolated muscle groups that are strength trained by the associated key exercises shown. The exercises are performed to more quickly define, tone, shape, and make more dense (thicken) your muscle fibers. They also will allow you to endure longer periods of work during your exercise program and later in your daily work tasks.

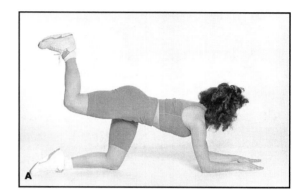

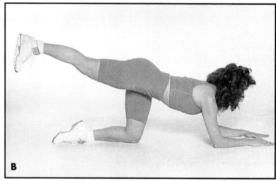

Figure 4.19. Thigh — Leg curls.

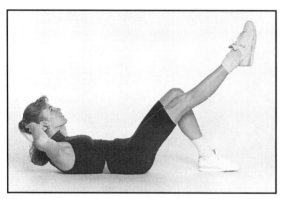

Figure 4.17. Abdomen — Curl-up variation.

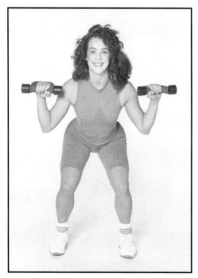

Figure 4.18. Buttocks — Squats.

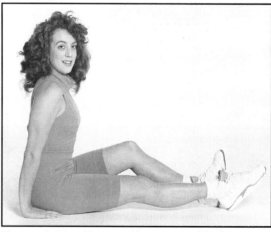

Figure 4.20. Shins — Alternating ankle flexion and extension.

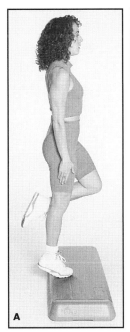 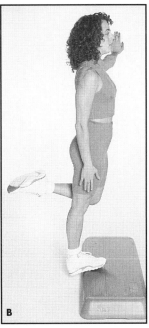

Figure 4.21. Calves — One-legged calf raise.

Because the focus is now on resistance work, which is better done when the body is thoroughly warmed, the time-frame becomes optional and is according to what you've prioritized time for in your workout session. If possible, you should plan approximately 10–20 minutes for strength training during aerobics class, using the following principles:

■ Precede and follow muscle strengthening exercises by stretching exercises specific for the muscles that are made to work against resistance. Any muscle group strengthened by exercise also should be stretched regularly to prevent abnormal contraction of resting length.[6]

■ Of key importance, stabilize your joints and your spine before beginning each exercise.

■ Perform each movement using a smooth, continuous, full range-of-motion action for the joint/muscle group involved, and keep the timing of the movement (usually slow) totally under your control. Ballistic (rapid or jerky) movements increase the risk of injury.

■ Take approximately 2 seconds to perform the overcoming-resistance (concentric) phase, and 2–4 seconds (i.e., at least the same time, or up to twice as long) during the release or lowering (eccentric) phase to return to the starting position of each exercise.[7]

■ Exhale during the lifting, overcoming-resistance-action move; inhale during the release or lowering and return. (Exception: During overhead pressing movements, inhale as you lift.)[8]

■ Engage in visualization and self-talk here. Plan your concentrated thoughts to accompany your lifting/exhale and lowering/inhale movements.

■ Follow the progressive resistance format. Begin with one to three sets of 8–12 repetitions for most exercises. (Exception: For abdominal work, begin your program by performing two sets of 15–30 repetitions per set). Select 8–10 exercises that condition the major muscle groups of your body for at least two of your aerobic sessions per week, if you have no other separate strength training program.

■ When you become jerky, are not smooth, continuous, and rhythmical in the move, and are not using the full range-of-motion possible around your joints, stop. You've completed your lower limit for that set. This lower limit becomes your baseline to which you attempt to add more repetitions as soon as possible.

■ Add resistance in increasingly greater increments (1–4 pounds if using hand weights, or thicker rubber if using bands/tubing). In the aerobics class setting, don't go over the 4-pound limit for hand-held weights if this is your choice of resistance equipment.

■ Do strength training of isolated muscle groups on an every-other-day basis. Your muscles need a day to recover, so don't incorporate a program to strength train with resistance (weights/bands/tubing) daily. As an alternative to this program, perform strength training exercises with resistance (weights/bands/tubing) for the upper half of your body one day and for the lower half of your body the next day. Thus, you are alternating the days that the muscles are strength training.

■ Allow brief rest periods between bouts of vigorous exercises. The time-frame for rest is defined as regaining a normal breathing pattern.

■ To incorporate variety into your program, try using all of the following forms of resistance:

1. Your own body (or parts) lifted and lowered against gravity as the weight resistance used, as in push-ups or curl-ups. (See Figures 4.13 and 4.17.) To progressively increase the resistance involved in lifting your body's weight against gravity, use a strategically placed free-weight (on the sternum for a curl-up, Figure 7.76, or between the shoulder blades for a push-up, and so on).

2. Hand-held weights (not wrist-weights) in controlled movement or placed on the body in the key locations to add weight resistance to the body part being lifted and lowered.

3. Rubber resistance bands, 9, 12, or 16 inches long, in widths of 1/4 to 1½ inches. The length and width is selected according to whether it is an upper or a lower body exercise, and your current strength fitness level in the muscle group being trained.

4. Rubber resistance tubing, approximately 3–4½ feet long, so you can adjust it according to your height in a range of light to heavy thickness that you select according to your current level of strength fitness.

5. All the above combined, using a step-bench in a level position, or in the gravity-assisted incline or decline positions. You will begin to realize, from the exercises

given in Chapter 7, that the possibilities for variety in your strength training segment are fun, exciting, inexpensive, and unlimited.

Options 3, 4, and 5 are illustrated in Figure 4.22. Following are the principles for using these unique pieces of equipment.

Using Resistance Bands and Tubing

The general directions for using either resistance bands or tubing are:

■ Select bands and tubing based on your fitness level.

■ Before each use, inspect the bands and tubing for nicks and tears that may arise from continued use.

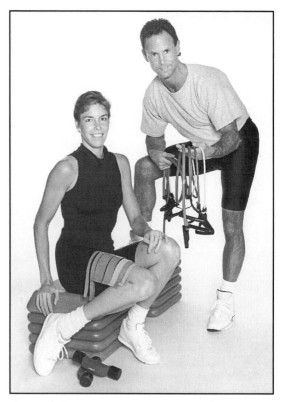

Figure 4.22. Various equipment to use for resistance.

■ Never, under any circumstances, tie pieces of band and tubing together.

■ Always exhibit proper body alignment and posture while exercising, as demonstrated in the following figures.

■ Keep your face turned slightly away from the direction of movement, for safety.

■ While performing single-limb upper body movements, always anchor the band between one hand and the thigh, hip, side, or shoulder, depending on the movement.

■ Always anchor the tubing under the ball of one foot or both feet, depending on your level of fitness and the desired amount of tension you wish to create.

■ Always control the bands and tubing, especially during the return phase of the movement. Do not let them control you.

■ Perform 8–10 repetitions of each exercise. When using one arm or one leg, switch sides so the same muscle group is worked an equal number of repetitions on the opposite side of the body. Be sure to work all muscular groups with equal intensity and repetitions at each session, to avoid muscular imbalance.[9]

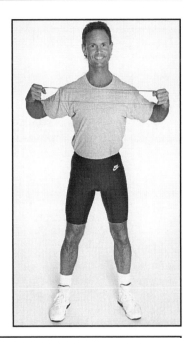

Figure 4.23. Using resistance bands for the upper body (deltoid press-away).

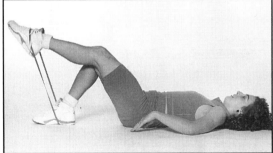

Figure 4.24. Using resistance bands for the lower body (leg extension for quadriceps).

Bands

Bands (Figures 4.23 and 4.24) are available in a variety of sizes to vary the intensity of your workout.[10] Suggested sizes:

■ **Beginner**
3/8" upper body (pink) or (light blue)
3/8" or 5/8" lower body

■ **Intermediate**
5/8" upper body (light blue)
5/8" lower body

■ **Advanced**
3/4" upper body (dark blue)
3/4" lower body

Tubing

Tubing also is available in a variety of sizes to vary the intensity of your workout.[11] Suggested sizes:

■ **Beginner**
Very light and light tubing (yellow or green)

■ **Intermediate**
Light and medium tubing (green or red)

■ **Advanced**
Heavy tubing (blue)

All of the tubing exercises described in Chapter 7 are designed for the beginner and intermediate exerciser. This means one foot will always be placed on the center of the tubing to create resistance. You can use the other foot to anchor the tubing if you like. Participants who want to create more resistance stand on the tubing with both feet. The wider you spread your feet, the more resistance you will create (Figures 4.25–4.27.[12]

Monitoring Your Progress

Record the exercises you perform, plus the number of sets, repetitions, and the type and amount of resistance you used with each exercise. Charting your progress gives you a visual blueprint for success and a means of continual motivation.

Begin this segment 3 of your program slowly, methodically, and in absolute control of the amount of resistance or weights you are using.

Strength-fitness training to more fully develop muscle strength and endurance is a long-term project[13] calling for a dedicated personal commitment of many hours, just as the programs of stretching for flexibility improvement and aerobics for aerobic capacity improvement are. All fitness programs are for life.

4 Cool-Down, Flexibility Training, and Relaxation

Gradual Cool-Down

The purpose of a planned cool-down portion of your hour is to give your body time to readjust to the pre-activity state in which you began. This will ease the gradual process of returning the large quantity of blood that is now in your working muscles, primarily in your arms and legs, back toward your head and trunk, brain, and other vital organs. Abruptly stopping a highly

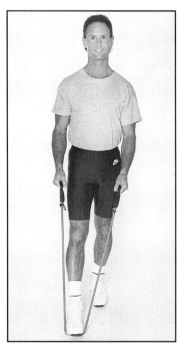

Figure 4.25. Beginner — Place one foot on tubing.

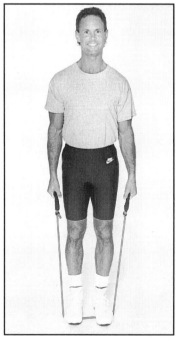

Figure 4.26. Intermediate — Place both feet on tubing.

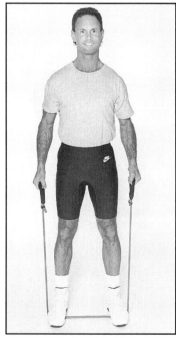

Figure 4.27. Advanced — Spread feet on tubing.

strenuous activity session may cause the blood (primarily in your legs) to pool, or stay in the extremities. This will occur because the veins of the legs are not being forcefully squeezed now by strenuously working leg muscles.

The result of pooling can cause cramping, nausea, dizziness, and fainting, because the needed quantity of oxygen and blood is not being delivered to the brain and other vital organs.

Your ability to recover from exertion usually will determine how long your cool-down period will have to be. A minimum of 5 to 10 minutes is essential, however, for two reasons:

■ To curtail profuse sweating.

■ To lower the heart rate to below 120 beats per minute.

These are two visible signs to monitor and achieve before concluding your exercise hour.

You'll begin your cooling down process by completely slowing down all large muscle activity. Tapering off your activity level can be done in various ways, such as slow-tempoed aerobics moves (Figure 4.28) or slow-paced walking. This

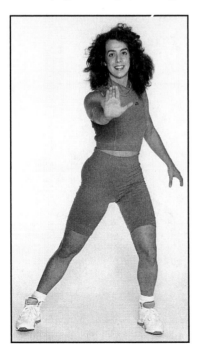

Figure 4.28. Cool-down with slow-tempoed aerobics moves.

segment begins the transition between the vigorous activity you've just completed and the flexibility training and relaxation you perform last.

Flexibility Training

Flexibility training, or stretching, is widely accepted as an effective means of increasing joint mobility, improving exercise performance, and reducing injuries.[14] Proper technique is essential, for the risks of injury may be significant if stretches are performed incorrectly.

Flexibility refers to the range-of-motion of a joint and its corresponding muscle groups. It is genetically influenced and highly specific and varies from joint to joint within an individual. Muscle, when stretched repeatedly, can be lengthened by approximately 20%,[15] whereas tendons can increase in length only about 2 to 3%.

Stretching programs follow the principle of Specific Adaptation to Imposed Demands (SAID), which states that an individual must slowly and progressively stretch the soft tissues around a joint to and slightly beyond the point of limitation, but not to the point of tearing.

At present, the two most widely accepted methods of stretching to improve flexibility are static and proprioceptive neuromuscular facilitatory (PNF) techniques. Both follow the philosophy that flexibility is increased and risk of injury is prevented when the muscle being stretched is as relaxed as possible.

Static stretching is slow, active stretching, with the position held at the joint extremes. The technique for executing stretching efficiently and safely is to ease gently into a controlled, stretched position and hold it as you gently press (Figure 4.29). You push or press to the point of tightness, "stretch pull" (not a pain, but a tight feeling) so you feel the muscle working. You continue to stretch a little beyond this point, without any motion. Then, mentally, you relax your mind and hold the position for approximately 15 seconds, allowing the muscle to also relax and feel heavier.[16] Continue to relax and slowly withdraw the stretch. Performing the same stretching on the opposite side of your body always follows.

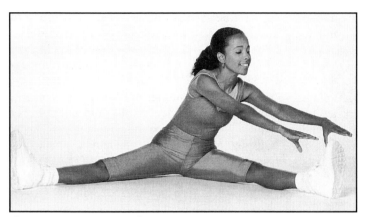

Figure 4.29. Static stretching.

At present, static stretching is considered to be one of the most effective methods of increasing flexibility, and research has shown that significant gains can be achieved with a training program of static stretching exercises. This type of continuous, long stretching produces greater flexibility with less possibility of injury, probably because it stretches the muscles under controlled conditions.

PNF stretching techniques, in which muscles are stretched progressively with intermittent isometric contractions, also offer an effective method of increasing flexibility and are used, like static stretches, when the muscles are warm. Two of the most commonly used modified PNF stretches are:

■ Contract-relax technique: In phase one, perform a 5–6 second maximum voluntary contraction in the muscle to be stretched. The contraction is isometric, because any motion is resisted. In phase two, relax, then stretch, the previously contracted muscle.

■ Agonist contract-relax technique: In phase one, maximally contract the muscle opposite the muscle to be stretched against resistance (a partner, the floor, or other immovable object) for 5–6 seconds. In phase two, relax the agonist muscle and stretch the antagonist muscle.[17]

An example of a forward PNF contract-relax exercise for the hamstrings and spinal extensors, shown in Figure 4.30, is performed with a partner's assistance. The position and actions are detailed.

■ Position: In a modified hurdler stretch position the performing partner lean forward to the point of limitation while keeping the back straight and the toes of the extended leg facing upward to correctly stretch the hamstrings.

■ Action: To begin the action, the performer pushes her back against the partner (contracting the spinal extensors) and pushes the extended leg against the floor (contracting the hamstrings) for a 6-second isometric contraction. The partner gently but firmly resists any movement.

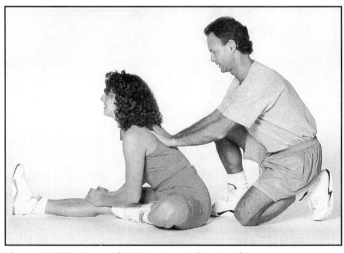

Figure 4.30. Forward PNF contract-relax stretching.

■ Action: After releasing the contraction, the performer stretches to a new point of limitation, holding a static stretch for 12 seconds or more, while the partner maintains a very light pressure on the performer's back.

Research has shown both static and PNF techniques for stretching to be effective. Both techniques can be used successfully to enhance flexibility.

Relaxation

Relaxation techniques complete your total physical fitness hour. These can be incorporated first during the stretching phase (Figure 4.31), to realize greater flexibility gains, and continued when stretching is completed, when an absence of muscle tension is established throughout the body.

When mental relaxation is initiated during the final stretching phase of the workout hour, the participant will focus on three key factors:

■ Mental images that are being constructed.

■ Self-talk accompanying each stretch and release (or contract-relax, according to which technique you use).

■ Mechanics of the breathing pattern.

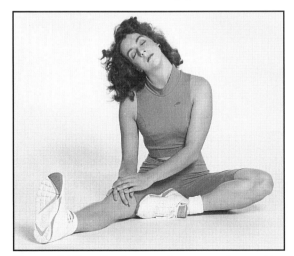

Figure 4.31. Combining relaxation with stretching segment.

Becoming highly motivated early on and then relaxing at the end requires a person to key into the same set of internal resources. The only difference between these two extremes is how you use these resources.

The mental images for relaxation initiated during the final stretching phase match the self-talk that accompanies it. The muscles being isolated and stretched are pictured and affirmed as becoming "wider, and longer, and warmer, and heavier."

The breathing pattern is sequenced with these pictures and affirmations. Begin with an 8-count deep breath initiated from deep down in the diaphragm area and inhaled through the nose. Hold this deep breath up to 8 seconds. As you slowly exhale through your pursed lips, formulate the pictures and affirmations: "wider-longer-warmer-heavier" . . . "wider-longer-warmer-heavier." Take about 16 seconds to slowly exhale and static stretch with these pictures and affirmations. Finally, as the stretch is slowly released and the muscle relaxed, begin another deep 8-count inhalation.

To match pictures and affirmations with the PNF stretching, mentally take apart the muscular actions that are transpiring and the time-frame suggested for each portion to take. Perform the exhalation breathing during the contractions.

Program Segments In Review

Outlined, the basic principles for the four key segments of an aerobics program workout session are:

Segment 1: Warm-Up

■ Active, rhythmic, limbering moves.

■ Slow, standing, static stretching.

■ Proper breathing technique throughout.

Segment 2: Aerobics

- Low-impact cardiovascular warm-up.
- Power low-impact with plyometrics.
- High- and low-impact.
- Power Low-impact with plyometrics.
- Low-impact cool-down.
- Post-aerobic stretching.

Segment 3: Strength Training and Calisthenics

- Focusing on isolated muscle groups — chest, arms, abdominals, buttocks, thighs, shins, and calves.
- Adding free weights, resistance bands, and tubing.

Segment 4: Cool-Down, Flexibility Training, and Relaxation

- Gradual cool-down moves.
- Flexibility training using static and PNF stretching.
- Relaxation techniques during and after final stretching moves.

Following an aerobics program such as this will provide you with a fun, safe, efficient, and complete workout session. If you prioritize this type of total physical fitness program into your schedule for a minimum of three days per week, you will have an excellent means of initially obtaining and then maintaining, your fitness for a lifetime.

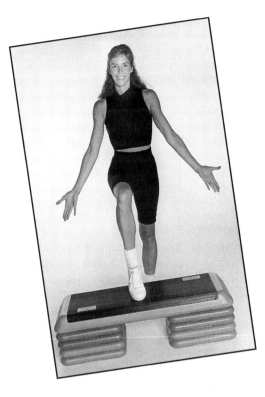

5

Enjoyment Through Aerobic Varieties

Motivation to stay with any fitness commitment will be enhanced by adding variety to your program when you need a change. Four unique possibilities to add to your aerobics program to help you solidify, or anchor, your fitness commitment are bench/step-training, interval aerobics/strength training involving the bench-step using tubing, pace-walking, and jumping rope.

BENCH/STEP-TRAINING PRINCIPLES

Bench/step training, or "step-training" currently is sweeping the aerobics and fitness industry with a new burst of enthusiasm and is the hottest aerobic trend of the 1990's. It is a relatively unexplored, new training modality with little research to date, so all the related common problems and injuries have not yet been fully assessed. To date, the following information and guidelines have been presented by various researchers promoting the activity and companies promoting products to use with the activity.[1, 2, 3, 4, 5]

Definitions and Benefits

Step-training is an exercise that involves stepping up and down on a platform or bench with a variety of upper torso movements added for further challenge. It has a variety of names — bench or step aerobics, bench- or step-training, bench-stepping, and stepping, to name just a few. All refer to the same activity.

The benefits are many. The key advantage to a step-training program is that it is primarily a *high-intensity activity* to promote cardiorespiratory fitness but *with low impact* for safety concerns. A vast majority of the moves can involve one foot supporting your weight, either on the bench platform or on the floor. Other benefits are:

- It is an excellent conditioning workout for the muscles of the legs, hips, and buttocks.

- Upper torso movements may provide conditioning for muscles of the arms, shoulders, chest, and back, and therefore a balanced and complete workout that strengthens and tones the entire body. This becomes especially you advance to using 1–4 lb. ts in a controlled manner, in your stepping moves.

■ As an effective cardiovascular workout, it has the aerobics benefits equal to running 7 mph, yet has the potentially low-impact equivalence of walking at a 3 mph pace.[6]

■ This workout is unique in its aerobics class versatility. The basic moves are simple, and by introducing various step patterns, all levels of participants can be challenged simultaneously. Regardless of gender or age, individuals can work at their own fitness level simply by doing less (or more) arm gestures, by adjusting the height of the bench, and by choosing to add or omit hand weights.

■ As an advanced, or skilled regular step-trainer with a high level of cardiovascular fitness, choose a 10″–12″ step (a 4″ platform plus a maximum of 4 support blocks on each end).

■ Participant height and leg length may dictate that a taller individual may prefer a bench step of 8″–12″.

■ Regardless of level of fitness or experience, you should not select a step height that allows the knee to flex less than 90 degrees (Figure 5.1) when the knee is weight-bearing. *If your knees advance beyond your toes as you step up, your platform is too high.*

An optional test for bench height is shown in Figure 5.2. Place one foot flat on top of the bench; allow a 3″ drop from the hip to knee for safe movement up to the top of the bench.

Choosing Your Bench Height

When selecting a bench height, consider the following factors:

■ As a beginner or novice who has not exercised regularly, or has limited coordination, or no experience in step-training, you initially should select a 4″ to 6″ bench. (For the 12″ bench shown in the chapter opening photo, this represents the basic 4″ platform, and at most one 2″ support block on each end.)

■ As an intermediate, or regular step-trainer with a "physically fit" level of cardiorespiratory fitness, choose an 8″–10″ step. (An 8″ bench equals a 4″ platform shown in the chapter opening and two 2″ support blocks. For a 10″ bench, add three 2″ support blocks.)

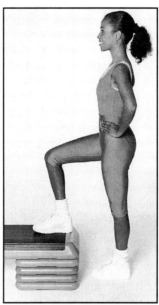

Figure 5.1. If your knees advance beyond your toes as you step up, your platform is too high.

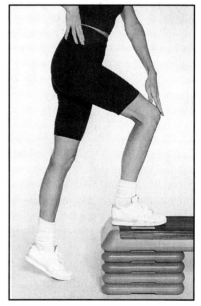

Figure 5.2. Allow a 3″ drop from the hip to knee.

Step To The Beat

Music plays a significant role, providing the underlying structure of a step-training program. The tempo of the music (measured as BPM — beats per minute) determines the speed and develops the progression of the movement performed.

Using music with a BPM of 118–125 is best. This will keep the movements controlled. Advanced workouts that follow all safety guidelines of alignment and technique may include tempos up to 135 BPM.

Listed below are class segments, with the suggested time durations and tempos of each.[7]

Duration/ mins.	Segment	BPM
10	I. Warm-Up	130–140
20–40	II. Aerobic Stepping &	118–120
3–5	Aerobic Cool-Down	118–120
10–15	III. Strength Training	120–130
5–10	IV. Stretching	<100

Body Alignment and Stepping Technique

Good posture is required for a safe, injury-free workout. Proper alignment and stepping technique are to:

■ Keep your back straight, head and chest up, shoulders back, abdomen tight, and buttocks tucked under hips, with eyes on the platform (Figure 5.3).

■ As much as possible, keep your shoulders aligned over your hips. Lean forward with the whole body. Don't bend from the hips or round the shoulders and lean forward or backward.

■ Step up lightly, making sure the whole foot lands on the platform, with the heel bearing your weight.

■ At the top, straighten your legs but don't lock your knees; keep them "soft."

■ As you step down, stay close to the platform. Land on the ball of the foot (Figure 5.4), then

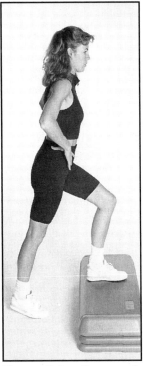 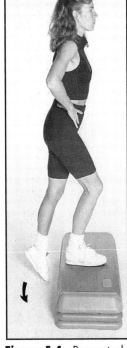

Figure 5.3. Proper technique for stepping up.

Figure 5.4. Proper technique for stepping down.

bring the heel down onto the floor, before taking the next step.

Step Technique Progression

Beginners should start on a 4″ bench, using no weights, at a moderate tempo for no more than 10 minutes per session. As you progress in skill and fitness level, the length of time stepping can be increased. When you can easily complete an entire session, the platform height can be raised, the music tempo can be increased, the arms can be used through a wider range-of-motion, and 1 to 4 lb. hand weights can be added.

Only one variable should be changed per session. Don't increase platform height and add weights at the same time. Increasing several variables at the same time doesn't allow your body time to adequately adapt to these changes and stressors.

Start with your hands on your hips, and concentrate on your feet and legs as your first priority. Once you've become proficient with the basic footwork skills and your fitness level has improved, increase the intensity of your program through your arm movements. This can include controlled complicated arm gestures *or* the use of hand weights.

The arm movements used with or without weights are those taken from the strength training programs that safely use long-and short-lever moves in a full range-of-motion action. All arm movements must move with the step pattern. This means arms go forward when stepping on the bench, back when stepping off, and up on a propulsion move. Think to use muscle more than momentum (i.e., control), and you will keep it a safer workout.

A Few Precautions

- Avoid excessive arm movements over your head.

- Maintain appropriate speed for safe and effective movement.

- Do not perform more than 8 counts (4 repeaters) on one leg at a time. Repeated foot impact without variation is potentially harmful.

- Do not pivot or twist the knee on the weight-bearing leg.

- Do not step up with your back toward the platform.

- If you are pregnant, check with your doctor before starting this program. If you are cleared by your doctor, make certain to keep your heart rate at 23 beats or below for a 10-second count. A step height of no more than 6 inches is recommended during pregnancy.

- If you feel faint or dizzy or if any exercise causes pain or severe discomfort, stop the exercise immediately but continue to move around.

- Maintain muscular balance by working opposing muscle groups equally (i.e., quads/hamstrings).

- Limit one person to a bench at a time.

- For the bench shown in the chapter opening photo, do not use more than four support blocks on each end of the platform.

Adding Hand-Held Weights to Stepping

Using 1–4 lb. hand-held weights in a step training program allows you to increase both exercise intensity for continual cardiovascular fitness gains and muscular strength and tonus, especially in the upper torso (Figure 5.5). The low-impact nature of step training, along with controlled stepping patterns performed at a moderate tempo, make it possible to safely use hand-held weights,[8] provided that you adhere to the

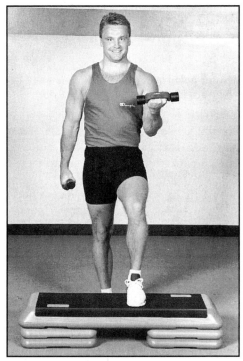

Figure 5.5. Hand-held weights can be used in conjunction with step training.

following safety precautions, and those previously mentioned.

1. Add hand weights, using 1 or 2 lb. weights, only after you are proficient at step training and when you have achieved an intermediate level of fitness.

2. Do not use hand weights if you:
   - Have high blood pressure.
   - Have a history of coronary disease.
   - Have low back pain.
   - Have arthritis.
   - Have other chronic or temporary orthopedic problems.
   - Are past the first trimester of pregnancy.
   - Are significantly overweight.

3. When you begin using light weights, use them for just one routine per session, and gradually build up your endurance. Start low and go slow.

4. Begin by using slow, small ranges-of-motion with short-lever, non-rotational arm movements, and never use flinging or uncontrolled movements.

5. Avoid maintaining arms at or above shoulder level for extended periods (i.e., overuse of tendons that stabilize the shoulder joint and unnecessary blood pressure elevation).

6. Avoid full-arm extension moves in short counts of music time.

7. Avoid using weights while performing propulsion steps.

8. Feel free to put down weights during your workout at any time. Place them safely under the bench or where you'll not accidentally step on them.

Adjusting Your Intensity

To decrease or increase your heart-rate pulse, try the following measures:

To Decrease

1. Do not use weights.
2. Keep hands on hips.
3. Lower bench height.
4. Perform movements only on floor.
5. Decrease music tempo.

To Increase

1. Make larger range-of-motion arm movements.
2. Add 2″ support blocks to bench height.
3. Add 1–4 lb. hand-held weights.
4. Increase music tempo.

Principles of Step Bench Using Tubing

Chapter 7 presents a variety of exercises using tubing in combination with the step bench, for either weight training alone, or for an *interval aerobics/strength training workout*. The key to the latter workout is incorporating 1-minute intervals of tubing exercises using the bench, with the body pressed into a "bent-knees" position on the action of the exercise. This position helps to keep the heart rate in the training zone during strength training and provides another safe, unique variety of exercises in your aerobics programming.

Bench/Step Training Summary

Incorporating a bench/step training program in your lifetime aerobics fitness plan has many advantages and benefits. It is a high-intensity exercise that sustains the training zone heart rate needed for the cardiorespiratory training effect to occur. Yet it is low-impact and safe, as one foot remains on the bench or the floor. Safety precautions include selecting the correct bench height, good body positioning and alignment, variety in technique to prevent overuse, and following the guidelines for incorporating arm gestures. Adding weights and resistance tubing can work together to establish an exciting new modality variety of aerobics training. Chapter 7 presents the details of techniques to use.

PACE WALKING

Pace walking is probably the easiest of all aerobic options because it can be done anywhere with no need for equipment or another's direction. Because it takes three times as long to get the same aerobic benefits from walking as from running,[9] *time* is a key factor when planning variety. Exercise action taking 14 minutes or longer per mile is classified as *walking*, taking 9–12 minutes per mile is labeled *jogging*, and *running* is taking under 9 minutes per mile.[10]

Principles and techniques for pace walking are:

- Wear supportive walking or running shoes and loose, comfortable clothing.
- Walk with the heel of the shoe contacting the ground first (Figure 5.6), with a rolling action forward, continuing through the ball of the foot. Eliminate any tendency for a bobbing, up-and-down motion.
- Hold arms in a long-lever (relaxed-elbow) position, with a forward and backward controlled swinging motion to involve upper torso conditioning also.

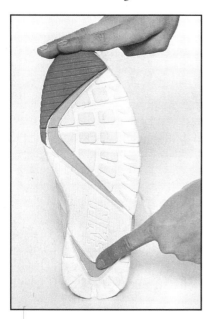

Figure 5.6. Walk with the heel of the shoe contacting the ground first.

- If weights are used, follow all the guidelines given earlier for using hand-held weights, with special attention to controlling your arm motions. Use very light weights, if any at all.
- Keep your posture erect at all times, and a relaxed lower back. Swing your hips freely forward and backward. Enjoy an easy, continuous breathing pattern.
- Follow all the aforementioned guidelines for aerobics programming, including adequate warm-up and cool-down.

The Level I Walking Program shown on Table 5.1 is a 10-week program. Remember to:

1. Warm-up and cool-down.
2. Walk briskly for at least 45 minutes, three to five times per week, to achieve maximum aerobic benefit from this program.[11]

JUMPING ROPE

Jumping rope is a strenuous activity that uses approximately three times more energy than leisure walking. This high-impact activity is not suited for everyone. Inactive individuals or those with joint or back problems should not participate in this form of aerobics. Others with exercise experience should have no problem.

The procedure involves the following:

- For jumping rope, use a rope of correct length, and preferably a giving surface upon which to jump. The correct length of rope is for it to reach your armpits (Figure 5.7), when held down tightly under your feet, with a few extra inches, or a handle, with which to hold the rope comfortably. If no handles are present, tape the ends or tie knots at the ends to prevent fraying. Among the variety of jump ropes on the market are beaded, licorice, leather, and cotton ropes. Beaded ropes and leather ropes are the best choice. Licorice (plastic) ropes get tangled more frequently,

TABLE 5.1   Level I — Walking Only*

Week	Session	Warm Up	Exercise	Warm Down	Goal (Distance)
1	1	yes	15-20'	yes	0.5 to 0.8 mi.
	2	yes	15-20'	yes	0.9 to 1.0 mi.
	3	yes	20'	yes	0.9 to 1.0 mi.
2	4	yes	20'	yes	0.9 to 1.0 mi.
	5	yes	24'	yes	1.1 to 1.2 mi.
	6	yes	24'	yes	1.1 to 1.2 mi.
3	7	yes	28'	yes	1.3 to 1.4 mi.
	8	yes	28'	yes	1.3 to 1.4 mi.
	9	yes	32'	yes	1.4 to 1.6 mi.
4	10	yes	32'	yes	1.4 to 1.6 mi.
	11	yes	36'	yes	1.7 to 1.8 mi.
	12	yes	36'	yes	1.7 to 1.8 mi.
5	13	yes	40'	yes	1.9 to 2.0 mi.
	14	yes	40'	yes	1.9 to 2.0 mi.
	15	yes	44'	yes	2.1 to 2.2 mi.
6	16	yes	48'	yes	2.3 to 2.4 mi.
	17	yes	48'	yes	2.3 to 2.4 mi.
	18	yes	48'	yes	2.3 to 2.4 mi.
7	19	yes	52'	yes	2.5 to 2.6 mi.
	20	yes	52'	yes	2.5 to 2.6 mi.
	21	yes	56'	yes	2.7 to 2.8 mi.
8	22	yes	56'	yes	2.7 to 2.8 mi.
	23	yes	60'	yes	2.9 to 3.0 mi.
	24	yes	60'	yes	2.9 to 3.0 mi.
9	25	yes	58'	yes	3.0 mi.
	26	yes	58'	yes	3.0 mi.
	27	yes	56'	yes	3.0 mi.
10	28	yes	56'	yes	3.0 mi.
	29	yes	54'	yes	3.0 mi.
	30	yes	54'	yes	3.0 mi.

*Program written by Dr. Richard Bowers, ACSM certified Program Director

and cotton ropes are rather difficult to use because they are so lightweight.

■ When you warm up, be sure to static stretch all the muscles of the leg, with special attention to the calf, heel cord, and shin areas.

■ Begin the aerobics segment with 6 minutes, progressing up to a 20-minute workout.

■ Restrict continuous jumping to 1-minute intervals at 120–140 revolutions per minute, which is a moderate pace. Alternate 1-minute segments with non-jumping low-impact aerobics such as marching or power walking. Music should range from 120–140 beats per minute also, to assist in timing and rhythm.

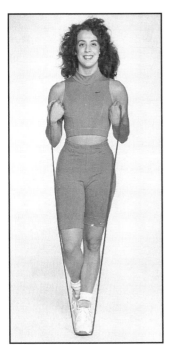

Figure 5.7.
Select correct
length of rope.

Alternate immediately to the other foot for the same number of steps.

2. Two feet at a time.

3. Jump with arm/rope crossed, followed by a one-footed or two-footed jump.

4. Hopscotch jump using a two-foot jump stride, one-foot jump, two-foot jump stride, alternate one-foot jump.

MONITORING YOUR PROGRESS

Take time immediately after each exercise session to record your progress and gains in a journal. Record any setbacks also. It will give you a visual blueprint on how successfully you are accomplishing a variety of short-term goals, and how you can do so again in the future. Include today's date, exercise varieties, time duration, short-term goal set, new achievement today, and your thoughts and feelings.

■ Jump low with "soft" knees for efficiency, and only high enough to clear the rope (less than 1 inch).

■ Use rate of perceived exertion (RPE) for monitoring your intensity because it allows you to monitor minute-to-minute how you feel.

■ Be sure to include a 5–10 minute cool-down, with non-jumping low-impact moves, and flexibility and relaxation for 5 minutes, doing static stretching for the leg muscles.[12]

Try a variety of rope-jumping skills (Figure 5.8):

1. One foot and then the other. If you jump on only one foot, don't do more than four repetitions on the same foot.

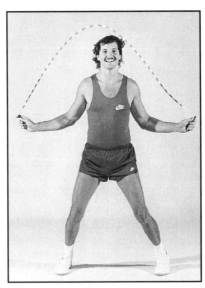
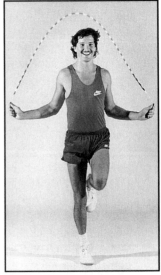

Figure 5.8. Variations on basic rope-jumping.

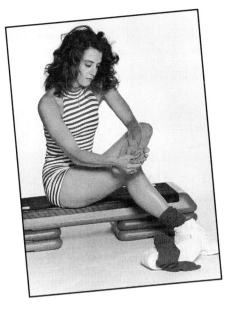

6

Safety First: Guidelines and Good Positioning

The enjoyment found in a new activity can bring longlasting benefits to your total wellness and vitality. Positive gains can be achieved by following the principles for safe, efficient movement. An element of risk is associated with all physical activities, however. By taking proper preventive measures, problems and injuries can be avoided. The following concerns are detailed to increase your awareness of the more common program-related problems you may incur. Understanding prevention is the key to a safe program.

SENSIBLE TRAINING

Planned self-discipline is required to become and stay physically fit, but the dividends of wellness and vitality are well worth it. Some tips in sensible training are:

1. Progress gradually in your sessions.

2. Remember to warm up and cool down.

3. Progress from easy to advanced both in the stretches and in the aerobic combinations.

4. Do not perform to the point of exhaustion. Learn to read your body signs. You're going to perspire and you're going to tire a little. With an effective aerobics program, you may encounter some initial, slight, temporary discomfort.

5. Pace yourself. For example, after engaging in several aerobic exercise movements or a complete step-training routine, you may be short of breath, but this should subside within minutes after the activity. If it doesn't subside, you've worked too hard.

6. If you are unsure about a specific discomfort or pain, ask a reliable person (such as your doctor) before continuing with activity.

SIGNS OF OVEREXERTION

Monitoring your pulse helps determine how hard to exercise your body, but you also need to be aware of your own bodily signs. Signs of overexertion are:

- Severe breathlessness.

- Poor heart rate response (continually monitoring too high an exercising heart rate that does not drop significantly after one minute of recovery, or final heart rate not below 120 beats per minute after five minutes of cooldown.

- Undue fatigue during exercise and inability to recover from a workout later in the day.

- Inability to sleep at night.

■ Persistent, severe muscle soreness. (The type of muscle soreness to guard against is not immediate but becomes apparent after 24-48 hours).

■ Nausea, feeling faint, dizziness.

■ Tightness or pains in the chest.

These symptoms do not mean you should not exercise; rather, they suggest a reduced level of activity until you develop the capacity to handle more intense workouts. An exercise program should be undertaken cautiously, and the frequency, intensity and duration of each session increased gradually.

If you have any of the following symptoms, ease down to a slow walk, sit with your head between your knees, or lie down on your back and elevate your feet. This will help the blood move to your head more readily and carry the needed oxygen to your brain. If any of these symptoms persist, contact your doctor.

NOTE: *Seek medical advice immediately and before the next exercise session if any of the following symptoms occur:*

---

1. Abnormal heart action

   ■ Irregular pulse.

   ■ Fluttering, jumping, or palpitations in chest or throat.

   ■ Sudden burst of rapid heartbeats.

   ■ Sudden, very slow pulse when a moment before it had been on target (immediate or delayed).

2. Pain or pressure in the center of the chest or the arm or throat precipitated by exercise or following exercise (immediate or delayed).

3. Dizziness, light headedness, sudden incoordination, confusion, cold sweat, glassy stare, pallor, blueness, or fainting (immediate).

   Do not try to cool down. Stop exercise and lie down with your feet elevated, or put your head down between your legs until the symptoms pass.[1]

VARIABLES

Numerous variables comprise an aerobics program. These include presence of illness, infection, or injury; lack of exercise for a while; location and environment; and shoe selection.

Presence of Illness, Infection, or Injury

The presence of illness, infection, or injury will show up in your "thermometer" of fitness, your pulse. It will be higher at rest and will escalate to the training zone with less than your usual effort. In that event, take it easy and decide whether to mentally "walk" through your program to maintain your discipline of exercising or to curtail exercise until you're completely well again.

Missing a While?

If you have missed aerobic exercise for a time, return to it slowly. When you miss activity several times, you will need to start more cautiously, as though beginning a new program. For example, you may have a bout of flu and are unable to exercise for a week. When you are able to exercise again, do *not* plan to start where you left off. You will need to return cautiously to the fitness level you were at before the illness.

Lenore Zohlman, a leading cardiologist in the U.S., has stated that you will lose approximately half of your fitness program gains after just 5 weeks if you discontinue your program totally. After 10 weeks of no aerobic activity, you will have lost most of your fitness gains.[2] Whenever a circumstance curtails your program, return slowly and systematically.

Location and Environment

Select a convenient and physiologically safe location for your workouts. Choose a *wood*-based floor or an area carpeted with flat nap and thick padding. (Carpeted surfaces tend to make lateral moves and turns risky, however.) Try not to exercise on concrete, as it has no "give" or buoyancy. Concrete adds unnecessary stress on your legs and feet.

> A resilient floor should be selected for exercise that involves repeated foot impacts. If such a surface is not available, the exercise routines should be modified to ensure that the feet remain close to the floor throughout the program (low-impact exercises).[3]

If relative humidity is high and temperature is 85° (room or outside) curtail your aerobic dance-exercise or step-training programs. Seek out another option, such as aerobic swimming in a cool-air environment.

For aerobic exercise, a cold environment doesn't matter as long as you thoroughly protect yourself, especially your air passages (at 40° and below, cover your air passages). Heat, however, does matter. Heat stress injuries can occur if you abandon caution.

SHOE SELECTION

The shoes you wear constitute one of your major concerns. When you jump or run, you place three to six times more force on your feet than when you are stationary. If you weigh 125 pounds, this means you are placing 375 to 750 pounds of pressure on your feet with each jump or run. Your body can withstand the stress of exercise better if you wear shoes that "shock-absorb" this pressure, or exercise on a surface with a giving quality. Select a shoe that totally supports your foot for the exercise modality you choose to engage in regularly. The following criteria and Table 6.1[4] give specific guidelines for personalizing your shoe selection.

- Inquire about midsole composition. For durability and performance, select shoes made from either compression-molded ethyl vinyl acetate (EVA) or polyurethane.

- Stay with the same brand and model of shoe you are currently replacing if it has been satisfactory.

- Do not allow yourself to be forced or pressured into buying a shoe that does not feel comfortable.

- Replace a single pair of shoes worn at least four days per week for any fitness-related activity about every four months. If the shoes have a polyurethane midsole, the wear may be extended up to six months. If they have a standard, open-cell EVA midsole, they may last only three months.

- Examine the inside of the shoe as well as the insole. Shoes with removable insoles are preferable because they tend to be better cushioned and allow the fit of a custom foot orthotic, if needed.[5]

- Nylon uppers are cooler than leather uppers. If you prefer an all-leather shoe, be sure it has ventilation holes on the top and sides. Extra design leather or suede along the ball-edge of the foot area (toes) provides longer shoe life.

- Choose a shoe that has a sole with a relatively smooth tread[6] and of white rubber, designed for aerobic dance-exercise or court use. Jogging shoes with black rubber soles, designed for road and track running and with rubber triangles, squares, circles, or thick waves provide excellent forward movement, but because aerobic dance-exercise consists of forward, backward, and lateral movement, this is not the best choice of shoe sole.

> The rough treads of most running shoes can be hazardous during aerobic dance-exercise as they can cause the feet to come to an abrupt halt each time they strike the floor. Thus, most shoes designed for running are unsuitable for aerobic dance.[7]

- If you have the tendency toward pronated ankles (lower leg bones do not sit directly on the ankle, as shown in Figure 6.1) do not select a wide heel flair of rubber. This heel flair will not only limit, to some extent, your lateral (sideward) movement, but it also will not provide the appropriate correction to avoid future possible injury to naturally weak ankles, as it does in jogging, which is all

TABLE 6.1. Personalizing Your Shoe Selection

IF YOU:	PICK A SHOE THAT:
are heavier or taller	has a firm, dense midsole, like polyurethane (PU)
are lighter or smaller	has a softer midsole, like compression-molded ethyl vinyl acetate (EVA).
have a high arch	is well-cushioned and soft.
have a flexible arch or flat foot	is firm and has motion-control features.

IF YOU HAVE HAD:	PICK A SHOE THAT:
stress fractures	is cushioned in the midsole and insole.
plantar fasciitis	is flexible and has a well-contoured insole with a prominent arch support.
ankle sprains	has a firm PU midsole with a 3/4"-high reinforced upper.
shin splints	has an elevated heel, plenty of cushion, and a contoured arch insole.
knee problems	has a firm sole with lateral reinforcement in the upper.

IF YOU PARTICIPATE IN:	YOU NEED:
aerobics/dance-exercise only	an aerobic-dance shoe or a cross trainer. If you have had arch or heel problems, choose an aerobics shoe because it is more flexible.
weight training, stair climbing* and stationary biking	a cross trainer.
aerobics/dance-exercise, weight training, stair climbing and biking	a cross trainer or aerobics shoe with a PU midsole.
aerobics/dance-exercise and running	an aerobics shoe and a running shoe.
aerobics/dance-exercise and fitness walking	an aerobics shoe and either a walking shoe or a running shoe.

* Step training is included here.

From Douglas H. Richie, "How to Choose Shoes," *IDEA Today*, April 1991, p. 67.

forward movement. Pronation of ankles can best be corrected inside the shoe by means of:

■ an extra firm heel box.

■ raising the arch with a specifically designed wedge.

■ controlling the floor contact of various portions of the foot by means of a specially designed orthotic (prescribed corrective device for the foot, as shown in Figure 6.2).

Sports orthotics are devices that are custom-made by hand to specifically control the function of your unique foot. They are not arch supports.

Requiring several weeks of construction, they are shaped to closely *control your foot the entire time it is on the floor or ground.* The bones in your foot are moved so the muscles can function and adapt normally, decreasing or eliminating foot problems. The orthotics are made of an unbreakable, reinforced material and are worn inside your athletic shoe.[8]

A person doesn't have to live with the pain that structural imbalances cause, such as aching on the entire bottom of the foot from the forward movement of running or shin splints from the lateral movement of aerobics. Sports orthotics can be prescribed by a qualified specialist, such as a podiatrist.

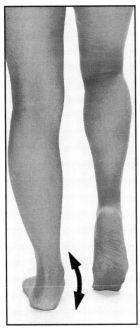

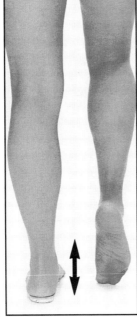

Figure 6.1. Pronation.   **Figure 6.2.** Correction with a sports orthotic.[8]

PROPER CLOTHING

Choosing what to wear for the environment in which you are exercising is important. Safety, comfort, and ease of movement are the criteria for aerobics apparel. You should dress in layers. A warm-up sweatsuit or jogging suit will assist in increasing the temperature of your arm and leg muscles during the warm-up portion. On very warm or highly humid and warm days, this, of course, is unnecessary. Cotton material is best, as it absorbs perspiration better than other fabrics. When cotton clothing becomes damp, the surrounding air causes the moisture to evaporate, and this cools the body.

During the routines, you want to be free to move in all directions and sweat freely, so you should wear as little as possible, especially when the temperature and relative humidity are high. Long, loose slacks should be avoided, as they can catch under the feet. The same is true for tight-fitting garments, as they restrict flexibility. The best advice for someone vigorously exercising is to keep clothing to a comfortable minimum. This allows unrestricted motion and facilitates loss of excessive body heat.[9]

Exercise apparel kept to a comfortable minimum is a guideline for all participants, to avoid heat stress injuries. Those who are overweight or obese are prime targets for overheating because they have a thick layer of fat tissue between internal organs and the outside layer of skin. It works like insulation and keeps internal heat in. The internal body systems may overheat and cause heat exhaustion or heat stroke. Therefore, don't try to "sweat" water pounds off by wearing lots of clothing or rubber-lined sweatsuits. Sweat and water loss are bodily cooling mechanisms and are not to be used as a measurement for weight loss because water is *not* fat!

To prevent friction in your shoes, wear cotton socks without wrinkles that will absorb sweat. This will help to keep your feet drier and free from blisters.

Cotton socks absorb sweat, so they keep your feet drier. They do not wrinkle, so they reduce friction and stave off blisters.

Finally, wearing a towel around the neck during exercise is contrary to all physiological principles. The major artery from the heart to the brain is located in the neck area, and it has to be free for cooling by exposure of the skin surface in that area to air.

FLUID INTAKE

Water is the principal means of transporting heat (and substances) within the body. In warm environments (meaning within a room or a geographical location), it is the *only* means of dispersing body heat. This is accomplished by the evaporation of released perspiration on the surface of the skin. When the room air contacts the sweat, the skin surface is cooled, and the cooling is then conducted internally. Production of body heat greatly increases during physical exercise.

Unless water for perspiration is available, body temperature increases beyond normal, causing over-heating. When fluid loss exceeds supply, dehydration follows, with an accompanying limited ability to exercise. When dehydration occurs, even modest physical activity causes the heart rate and body temperature to increase. When the water loss is approximately 5% of the total body water, evidence of heat exhaustion may become apparent, and when losses are 10%, the condition may soon lead to heat stroke, which is fatal unless attended to immediately (through an ice bath submersion).

Fluid intake must be increased to maintain fluid balance as the work level and environmental temperature increase.[10]

Because there is no basis for restricting water intake during aerobics and no evidence that humans can adapt or be trained to tolerate water intake lower than daily losses, you should replace water loss by continuous daily fluid intake. A few guidelines to facilitate water balance are:

1. Drink plenty of liquids at least 20 minutes before beginning an aerobics hour. Frequent, small intake of fluid throughout the day is best.

2. If you have been drinking plenty of water prior to aerobic sessions, you probably will not need to drink water during the hour (room temperature and humidity are the variables that usually determine this). If you get thirsty during the hour, however, drink water. Your thirst mechanism is a late sign that you need water, so don't ignore it!

3. After an aerobics hour, relax and sit with a tall glass of ice water or an inexpensive, home-made electrolyte ("sports drink") solution. This will provide immediate rehydration and is a pleasant way to conclude your session.

"Homemade" electrolyte solution[11]

1 qt. frozen reconstituted orange juice
3 qts. water
1/2 tsp. salt

Deliberate dehydration (by loading on the clothes and promoting profuse sweating), of course, is not an acceptable method for weight control. This will cause a temporary loss of weight, which is rapidly regained by rehydration. Loss of weight should be only body fat, not water or protein.

4. Many "sports beverages" are promoted as sources of available sodium, potassium, and sugar. Replacement needs for sodium and potassium can be met much better through a diet that contains a variety of foods and supplies these and other nutrients, including proper amounts of water. If the exerciser uses any of the sports beverages or commercial preparations, they should be diluted with water to decrease the concentration of sugar and thus decrease the time the fluid stays in the stomach. Recommended dilutions are given in Table 6.2.[12]

TABLE 6.2. Dilution of Replacement Fluids

Fruit juices	1 part juice; 3 parts water
Soft drinks	1 part soda; 3 parts water
Vegetable juices	1 part juice; 1 part water
Gatorade®	1 part drink; 1 part water
Pripps Pluss®	1 part drink; 3 parts water
Quickick® (orange flavor)	1 part drink; 3 parts water

But remember — water is the best replacement fluid.

COMMON INJURIES

Blisters

Blisters arise in seconds and take days to heal. Even a small blister that goes untreated will bother your workout. The best advice is to do everything you can to prevent them from forming.

Blisters are caused by friction as the surface of the shoe rubs against the skin of the foot. Shoes should fit well, not too loose and not too tight. To help prevent blisters, one tip is to lubricate the trouble spot with petroleum jelly before you put your shoes on for another fitness session. If you sweat a lot, powder your feet also. Because improper-fitting shoes are the culprit, be sure to do a few exertive moves in your local shoe store to size up comfort *in motion* before purchasing the shoes.

If you get a water blister, care for it as follows:

- Gently scrub the area with soap and water to thoroughly clean it.
- Gently swab with alcohol or a surgical preparation.
- Make two incisions at the outer edges of the blister. Slowly press out the superficial fluid.
- Apply ointment or first-aid cream.
- Bandage until healed completely.

If you get a blood blister, care for it as follows:

- Ice the area.
- Do not puncture. The chance of infection is great, as it connects with the circulatory system.
- Place a "donut"-type compress around the blister until it is reabsorbed and completely healed.

Bunions

A bunion is a large, bony protuberance on the outside of the big toe that indicates joint inflammation. The main causes of bunions are overpronation and faulty foot structure. Seek correction from a podiatrist.

Muscle Cramps

A cramp is a painful spasm of muscle. Cramping may occur during or following a vigorous exercise session. It is the result of two different phenomena. Muscle cramping *during* an exercise session primarily reflects an electrolyte and fluid imbalance in your system.[13] Electrolytes are sodium, calcium, chloride, potassium, and magnesium. Cramping occurs primarily because you have not, with regularity, properly replaced your water intake as you condition and train.

If a person has lost a lot of water through perspiration (eight or more pounds of water), replacement of those elements may be obtained by drinking, in solution (never in tablet form), a substance that replaces them. With moderate sweating and water loss, regular, daily water intake and proper diet will replace the needed fluids and electrolyte elements and do much to eliminate this type of cramping.

The most common cramps associated with exercise are those occurring in the *24 hours after* exercise, especially after having gone to bed or after a sudden movement. These cramps (post-exercise) are not associated with electrolyte imbalance.[14] They are believed to be caused by muscle fiber swelling, agitating the (peripheral) nerves servicing the muscle tissue. If these cramps are frequent and severe, the treatment prescribed, may be .2 grams of quinine sulfate.

Immediate relief for either type of cramping is to static stretch in the exact opposite direction for a few moments.

Muscle Soreness

Two types of pain are associated with severe muscular exercise: (a) pain during and immediately after exercise, which may persist for several hours, and (b) localized soreness that usually does not appear for 24 to 48 hours. The first is associated with metabolic wastes on pain receptors, the second with torn muscle fibers or connective tissue.[15] The first type need not cause great concern; it presents no lasting problems. The delayed type requires attention in the form of a more adequate warm-up and cool-down stretching program and incorporation of concluding strength activities.

Gradual, sensible muscle use during exercise is the best prevention.

Muscle, Tendon, and Joint Injuries

For *muscle strains or sprains*, you ICE (ice, compress, and elevate). Injuries are iced (or cold whirlpools are administered) to inhibit swelling and promote healing by making the body internally (rather than at the surface) supply more blood to the affected deep-problem area. The body forces more blood to come to the area when cold applications are applied by making the body work harder pumping away the old cells and pumping in fresh oxygen and nutrients to begin the repair process at the deep site rather than at the surface skin area.

Ice applications are administered two times a day for about 20 minutes. When the affected area no longer is warm to the touch (using the back of your hand) but seems to be the same temperature as the surrounding area, ice compresses can be stopped.

When heat is applied, it brings an increase of blood to the skin surface, but it doesn't make the body work hard at all, on its own, to pump in a fresh supply of oxygen and nutrients to the deep affected area. The less comfortable application of ice will hasten the repair process.

Achilles tendonitis is an inflammation of the thick tendon that connects the heel to the calf muscle. This injury results from wearing shoes with inadequately thick heels or that for some other reason do not provide a proper cushion for the foot. Biomechanical problems such as the following aggravate the situation: bowed legs, tight hamstrings and calves, high-arched rigid feet, overpronation, and excessive toe-running.

Adequate heel-cord stretching helps prevent Achilles tendonitis. As aggravation of this problem can cause a serious and permanent condition, the affected person should not continue to exercise with the pain.

Shin Splints

The most frequent injury to new aerobics enthusiasts is shin splints. It is signaled by pain on the front and inside of the lower leg (Figure 6.3). Although it is an affliction common in runners, this malady can affect anyone who engages in physical activity using the legs. Most cases of shin splints occur in the *beginning* of an exercise program because the lower leg muscles are weak.

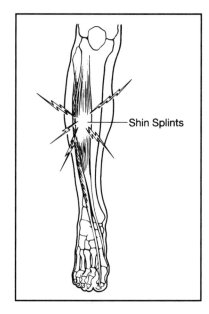

Figure 6.3.
Shin splints.

Jumping and running activities cause the leg muscles in the back of the leg to develop and become stronger while the leg muscles in front develop only slightly. This muscle imbalance can cause shin splints if it is not treated correctly.[16] When the strength of one muscle or muscle group is disproportionate to that of the antagonist(s) for that muscle or group, the weaker muscle should be strengthened to restore balance around the joint.[17]

Preventive measures include light, flexible shoes with good arch support. Stretching before and after physical activity also helps the muscles absorb shock. Track running should be avoided as the repeated turns put great stress on the lower leg. Performing a stretch using three repetitions of straight-leg and bent-knee wall leans for 20 seconds may help alleviate the problem (Figure 6.4). Another preventive measure is to develop the strength of the anterior lower leg area. This can be accomplished by performing an exercise such as the lower-leg flexor, which uses resistance/rubber tubing. Sit tall with your legs together in front of you and place the center of the tubing under the toes of your shoes. Place your hands comfortably in front of the abdomen and don't move them during the exercise. Slowly

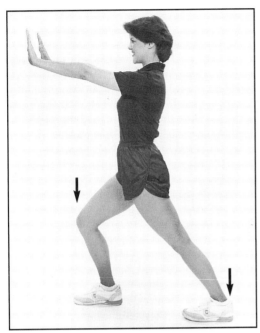

Figure 6.4. Shin splint relief.

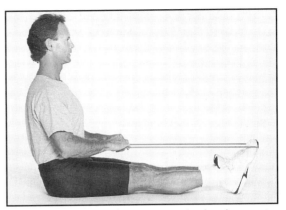

Figure 6.5. Strength exercise to develop the anterior lower leg muscles, **down** position.

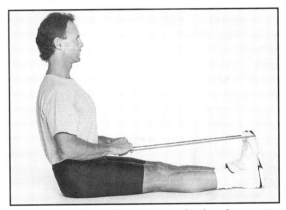

Figure 6.6. Strength exercise to develop the anterior lower leg muscles, **up** position.

point your toes down and toward the wall in front of you (Figure 6.5) and hold 15 seconds. Relax a few seconds, then flex your feet at the ankle and draw your toes up tightly toward your knees (Figure 6.6) and hold 15 seconds. Repeat entire exercise for several minutes. This can be done one leg at a time or both feet working together, simultaneously.

Of utmost importance in caring for shin splints are *rest and immediate icing* in the area of tenderness. The icing should be for 8–10 continuous minutes, while gently massaging the problem area. Later in the day, a second gentle ice massage for the same time duration should begin to give the desired relief. Continue this procedure for several days. You'll be amazed how quickly you heal within one week.

If icing, rest, aspirin (four to six per day), strengthening, and stretching do not create relief within 10 days, see a physician to rule out more serious conditions such as stress fractures, structural imbalances that might require orthotics, or anterior compartment syndrome.[18]

DRUG USE

As many as half of all heart attack deaths may occur because of "electrical failure," not "pump failure," of the heart. People with adequate amounts of heart muscle die because their heart's electrical signals go out of sync; the muscle then twitches chaotically and can no longer pump blood. Known as *ventricular fibrillation*, this rhythm disturbance is deadly if it cannot be reversed within minutes.[19] The drug-related deaths of superstar athletes in recent years by cocaine intoxication is directly related to this phenomenon.

SEEK THE PROFESSIONALS

Understanding the cause and effect will help prevent problems or injuries during the quest for fitness. Whenever problems or injuries do occur, you should seek out answers from qualified professionals — medical doctors, sports medicine specialists and physiologists, or athletic trainers.

Follow the diet, exercise, and mental training programs promoted by *scientific professionals*. Read and believe authors whose credentials are impressive in the various fields of total fitness and who publish their researched findings in *professional journals*. In this way, you have access to the most accurate, up-to-date knowledge available, and a more safe, fun way to good health.

POSTURE: GOOD POSITIONING UNDERLIES ALL MOVEMENT

Probably the reason to include posture information in an aerobics course is to *save your back!* To ensure that you are exercising in the *safest* possible fashion, you must understand good postural techniques, regardless of the activity. Poor posture is illustrated by Figure 6.7. Correct posture is shown in Figure 6.8.

The Mechanics

The downward pressure of gravity applied to the bones of the upright, balanced skeleton tends to cause it to buckle at three principal points: hip, knee, and ankle. Because the body weight is largely in front of the spinal column, the body tends to fall forward. To counteract these tendencies toward buckling and falling forward, five muscles or muscle groups are anti-gravity in nature, allowing for an upright, balanced skeleton. The anti-gravity muscle groups responsible for holding us erect are located in the:

- back, along with spinal column
- abdomen

- buttocks
- front of the thighs
- calves.

To develop good posture, the position of the spine, pelvic girdle, and hip joints (which act as the main hinges of the body) are to be controlled. This is done primarily by the five muscle groups. *How* you control them determines posture.

Balanced Static Posture

A balanced standing posture is established when:

- The head and stretched neck are balanced on top of the spine and centered above the shoulders, keeping the chin parallel to the floor.
- The shoulders are pulled back and down (in a relaxed position).
- The chest and rib cage are raised up.
- The abdominal muscles are pulled in and up, under the rib cage.

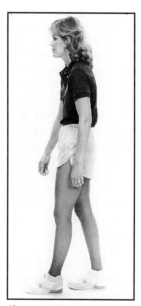

Figure 6.7.
Poor posture.

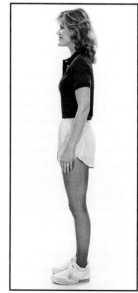

Figure 6.8.
Correct posture.

- The pelvic girdle is pulled down and under, tightening the buttocks. The pelvis rests on the two thigh bones balanced over two arched feet.

- The knees are relaxed. Locking the knees in a hyperextended position causes imbalance and increases susceptibility to knee injury.

- The weight is distributed equally on both feet while standing with the feet parallel and toes pointing forward, taking the weight on the outer half of the feet.

- The arms are relaxed.

Poor Posture

If any segment is out of body alignment, weight distribution will be uneven over the base of support and puts unnecessary strain on muscles, bones, and joints. This soon causes fatigue.

Poor posture is a habit that can be changed but it takes time, for it is a habit that has been a part of a person for a long time (Figure 6.9).

Most muscles are in pairs. If a muscle is constantly shortened, its opposing muscle lengthens and becomes weak from disuse. Therefore, stretching (lengthening) one set of muscles while simultaneously contracting (shortening) the opposing set of muscles, *and then repeating vice versa*, will strengthen both (especially if additional weight resistance is used).

With this information, you can understand why stretching and strengthening the muscles will lead to improved posture. If your body is to move freely, every muscle has to be able to shorten or lengthen in either a strong, quick manner or a slow, relaxed manner. Fully understanding the principles of stretching and of strength-training will assist you further in understanding and obtaining good posture goals.

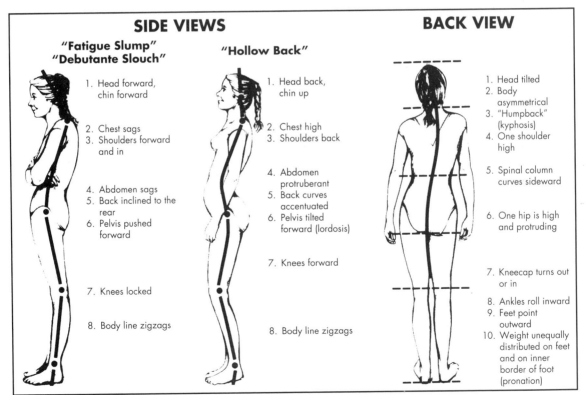

Figure 6.9. Characteristics of poor posture.

Efficient Positions

If you now have poor posture during aerobic movement activities, you will need to re-educate your neuromuscular system. This takes patience, persistence, and a sincere desire to want to improve both your appearance and the efficiency of your body.

If you were born free from hereditary or congenital deformities, you *can* obtain good posture (Figure 6.10). It's all a matter of:

- understanding balanced postures.
- developing a kinesthetic (sensory) awareness of your body positions during all movement.
- developing strong, yet relaxed, muscles and flexible joints.
- desiring to obtain good posture.
- discipline to continue what you have learned.

As you understand correct technique, challenge yourself to try using these positions in every total fitness component of your program, (stretching, aerobics, and strength-training exercises). At first you'll be "thinking through" the activity, but with persistent practice and desire, you can exchange any former faulty habits for safe, more complimentary ones.

If you can attain a balanced standing posture, you've mastered this task already.

Dynamic Posture

Performing the aerobics or step-training gesture and step patterns will require you to take a different body position, or posture, than when you are standing stationary and poised. You are dynamically preparing to move in some direction through space (forward, backward, laterally, up, down). While preparing to move through space, the broader your base of support, the lower your center of gravity (weight center) becomes. This allows for better balance so you can move quickly and more efficiently in any direction.

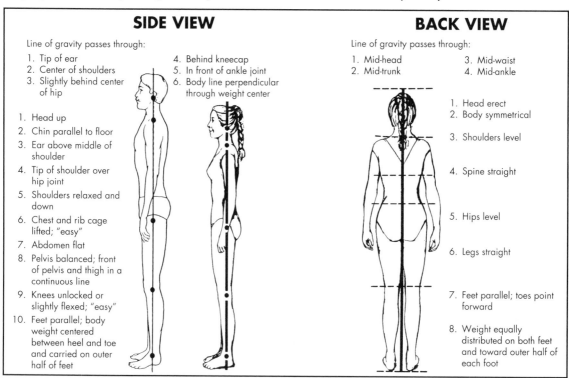

SIDE VIEW

Line of gravity passes through:

1. Tip of ear
2. Center of shoulders
3. Slightly behind center of hip
4. Behind kneecap
5. In front of ankle joint
6. Body line perpendicular through weight center

1. Head up
2. Chin parallel to floor
3. Ear above middle of shoulder
4. Tip of shoulder over hip joint
5. Shoulders relaxed and down
6. Chest and rib cage lifted; "easy"
7. Abdomen flat
8. Pelvis balanced; front of pelvis and thigh in a continuous line
9. Knees unlocked or slightly flexed; "easy"
10. Feet parallel; body weight centered between heel and toe and carried on outer half of feet

BACK VIEW

Line of gravity passes through:

1. Mid-head
2. Mid-trunk
3. Mid-waist
4. Mid-ankle

1. Head erect
2. Body symmetrical
3. Shoulders level
4. Spine straight
5. Hips level
6. Legs straight
7. Feet parallel; toes point forward
8. Weight equally distributed on both feet and toward outer half of each foot

Figure 6.10. Characteristics of good posture.

Step Training Postures

Three common step training errors to avoid are illustrated in Figures 6.11, 6.13, and 6.15. The man is demonstrating incorrect postural techniques for each exercise. In Figures 6.12, 6.14, and 6.16, the woman is performing correctly.[20]

Hip/leg extension

Undesirable curve of the lower back with an excessive rear leg lift and forward body lean.

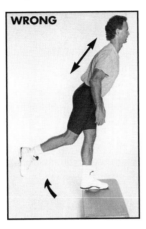

Figure 6.11.

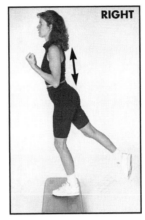

Stand tall on the platform and extend the rear lifting leg **back**, not up.

Figure 6.12.

Side step-out squats

Tendency to lean too far out to the side, which places too much stress on the knee.

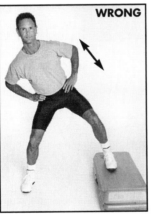

Figure 6.13.

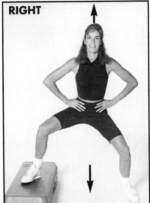

Balance your weight evenly, keeping center of gravity squarely within your legs.

Figure 6.14.

Step-back lunges from platform

Bending too far forward at the hip or having the leg reaching back in a locked-knee position. Heel should not be forced to the floor, as it may be too much dorsiflexion of the foot.

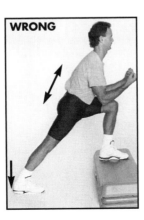

Figure 6.15.

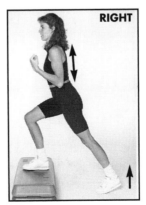

Keep body weight predominantly over the platform leg, and knee over toes. The leg reaching back should make floor contact, with knee slightly flexed. This reduces chance for joint trauma. Back heel is raised off the floor.

Figure 6.16.

Correct Lifting and Lowering

To protect your muscles and joints (especially the lower back) from undue strain or fatigue, proper technique in these areas *must* become second nature to you. Disciplined practice of correct techniques *now* will establish good habits for the rest of your life. The leg muscles are very strong, whereas the back muscles are relatively weak. All heavy lifting should be done by stabilizing the back in an erect position and making the legs provide the necessary power.

1. Get as close to the object as possible, using a forward-stride position. The object should be in front of you if you are using two hands (i.e., step-bench) or beside you if you are using one hand (i.e., luggage). Keep your back straight and your pelvis tucked, and bend at the hips, knees, and ankles to lower your body. Lower directly downward, only as much as necessary.

2. Both arms should be placed well under or around the weight center of the load. Lift vertically upward in a slow, steady movement by extending your leg muscles. Keep the object close to your weight center (Figure 6.17). Reverse the procedure to lower the object.

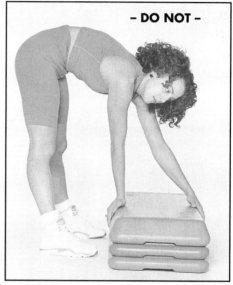

Figure 6.18. Incorrect lifting position.

Correct Carrying

1. Keep the object close to your weight center.

2. Separate the load when feasible, and carry half in each hand/arm (Figure 6.19).

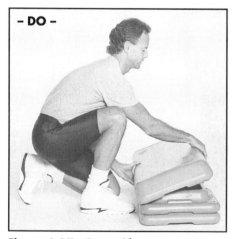

Figure 6.17. Correct lifting position.

Do not bend over from the hips (head low, buttocks high) and force your back muscles to lift the load (Figure 6.18).

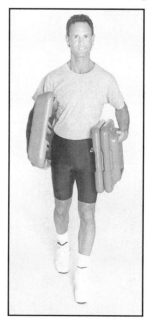

Figure 6.19. Correct carrying position.

Developing Postural Awareness Through Posture Exercises

Exercising the anti-gravity muscles is a fundamental part of any total physical fitness conditioning program. To develop and then maintain a good posture, these muscles have to be:

- *strong* enough to perform their functions.
- *flexible* enough to allow a variety of movement.
- *relaxed* enough to perform with ease.

Therefore, establishing a program of *strength* exercises for the abdomen, lower back, hip, thigh, and calf areas will help you to obtain a balanced pelvic alignment and provide the means for efficient and painless movement. And, as mentioned, each joint involved has to be flexible enough to permit the full range of movement possible from these groups of anti-gravity muscles so that any new position can be properly maintained. The following exercises will help you develop joint *flexibility* of the anti-gravity muscle groups needed to maintain correct postures. And, establishing a *program of relaxation* will assist with ease of performance, while moving or while motionless.

The *best* exercise you can do for yourself is both a physical and mental one: *Become aware of correct postural technique with every move you make.* Then practice this physical and mental conditioning constantly until it becomes a habit, until it becomes you.

Elbows Wide 'N Close

To understand the awareness of "space between shoulder blades" *contracted* and then *widely stretched*, keeping chest raised for either direction (see Figure 6.20):

1. Clasp your hands loosely behind you head (Figure 6.20a). Do not tightly lace fingers behind the neck. Pulling on the cervical spine is not a good body position. Keep your **elbows out and high**, shoulders down, and chin parallel to the floor. **4 counts.**

2. Exhale, and widen the space between your shoulder blades by bringing elbows **together** in front of your nose (Figure 6.20b). **Hold. 4 counts.**

3. Inhale, and return **elbows wide** to the sides (Figure 6.20a). **4 counts.**

4. Exhale and pull your elbows **up and back**, tightly contracting the space between your shoulder blades. **Hold. 4 counts.**

5. Inhale and return **elbows wide** to the sides (Figure 6.20a). **4 counts.**

6. For variety, repeat attempting to touch elbows together, first **in front of forehead** and **below the chin**, maintaining the good posture position.

Cues: "Elbows out and high, together, wide, up and back, wide."

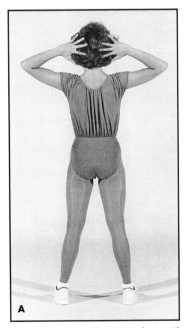
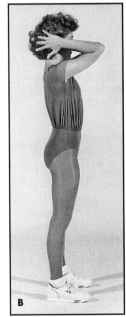

Figure 6.20. Elbows Wide 'N Close.

Rib Lifter

To establish awareness to the all-important position of "chest high" (and not sagging), this exercise (Figure 6.21) will help to isolate and stretch the intercostal (rib) muscles:

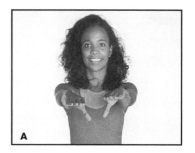

1. Stand in correct alignment, with your **arms forward** and **parallel** to the ground. Place your thumbs and index fingers of each hand together, hands forward, palms down (Figure 6.21a). **4 counts.**

2. Bend your elbows, bring your arms back, and place your palms parallel to the ground above your breast, with your **thumbs** snugly **under the armpits** and elbows held wide and parallel to the ground (Figure 6.21b). **4 counts.**

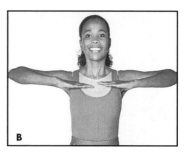

3. Without lifting your shoulders or bending forward, **lift your entire rib section as high as you can.** Breathe deeply, inhale, and exhale. **8 counts.**

4. Now **lift** your elbow high **and stretch** rib cage on the one side (Figure 6.21c). **4 counts.**

5. **Lower** raised elbow to shoulder level. **4 counts.**

6. Repeat with lifting and lowering of other elbow. **8 counts.**

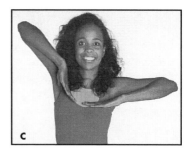

7. Repeat raising both together; lower. **8 counts.**

Figure 6.21. Rib Lifter.

Cues: Stand; thumbs under armpits; lift ribs and breathe; lift and stretch, lower; repeat other side; repeat both; lower.

For your total daily well-being, good posture must become important enough to you to be a lifelong endeavor. Are you sitting correctly while reading how to improve your posture?

Daily practice is required for it to become an integral part of you. Good posture is established only through *discipline*. Setting aside time to perform techniques and exercises to encourage good posture and develop strength and flexibility, accompanied by constant attention to posture throughout your daily living tasks, will make this become a reality. You can improve as you move — all day, every day — for this is where your total program for a fit physique begins!

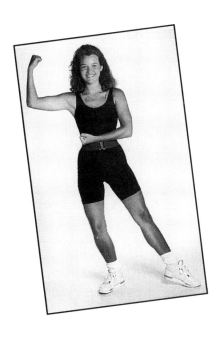

7

Program Techniques: Start to Finish

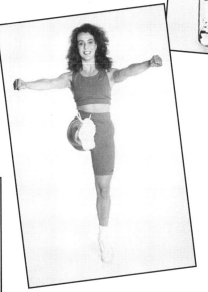

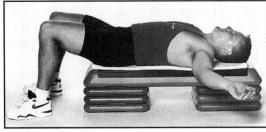

Complete background information needed to safely and efficiently enjoy an aerobics and step training exercise program has been established in the first six chapters. This chapter of aerobic techniques is a visual resource of exercise movement depicting basic steps and gestures for each of the four key program segments:

1. Warm-up
2. Aerobic exercise / step-training
3. Strength training
4. Cool-down / flexibility training / relaxation

The techniques are photographed and described by the "mirroring technique," in which the words and movement are to be done exactly as shown.

1. WARM-UP

The warm-up segment consists of active, low-level, rhythmic, limbering, standing, range-of-motion type of exercises for approximately 5 minutes, followed by 5 minutes of slow, sustained, static stretching from head to toe. Principles for each are described and shown in Chapter 4. The figure references in brackets throughout this chapter are a cross-reference to additional applicable exercises in other chapters.

■ ACTIVE, LOW-LEVEL, RHYTHMIC, LIMBERING, STANDING MOVES

Figures 7.1–7.2

Figure 7.1. Step-Touch

With big arm curl swings.

2 counts

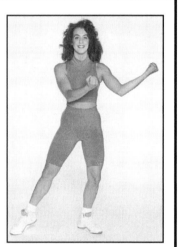

Figure 7.2. Step-Out Wide and Squat

Hold, side-clap, side-clap.

4 counts

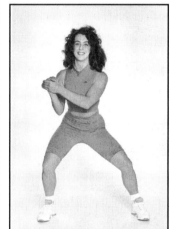

■ STATIC STRETCHING MOVES[1]

Figures [4.1–4.2; 4.11–4.13] 7.3–7.10

Figure 7.3. Shoulder Circles

Up, back, down, forward; or alternate, one at a time.

4 counts in each direction

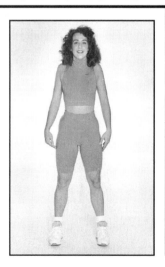

Figure 7.4. Arm Sweeps

Low and center; wide and palms up; raise, reach high.

8 counts

Reverse

8 counts

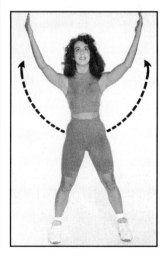

■ STATIC STRETCHING MOVES

Figure 7.5.
Chest

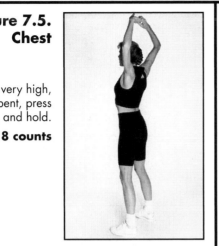

Grasp hands very high,
elbows bent, press
back, and hold.

8 counts

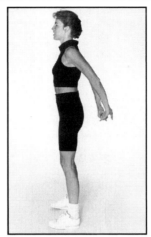

Figure 7.6.
Chest

Grasp hands low,
behind back, lift
and hold.

8 counts

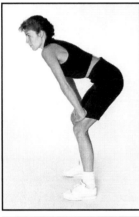

Figure 7.7.
Low Back

Feet apart, hands on
thighs; flatten back,
hold.

8 counts

Figure 7.8.
Low Back

Now round lower
back upward, contract
abdominals, tuck
buttocks under hips,
and hold.

8 counts

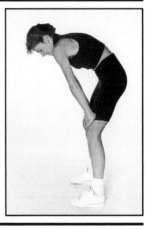

Figure 7.9.
Inner Thigh

Feet apart/toes
forward, shift
weight/hips right
(R), flex R knee over
R toe, and hold.

8/16 counts

Reverse.

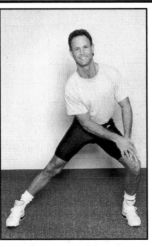

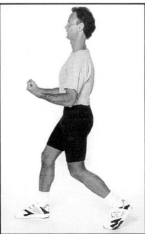

Figure 7.10.
Hip Flexors

Forward/back stride,
feet forward, fists at
waist; firmly tuck
buttocks under hips,
flexing knees/lower-
ing elbows, and hold.

8/16 counts

Reverse.

2. AEROBIC EXERCISE

Any activity that promotes the supply and use of oxygen using the criteria established in Chapter 2 can be performed during this 20–60 minute segment of time. This includes the pace walking and jumping rope detailed earlier, and the aerobics and step training presented here.

Aerobics   Figures [4.3–4.10], 7.11–7.36

■ LOW-IMPACT AEROBICS   Figures 7.11–7.18

Figure 7.11. Bounce 'n Hitch-Kick

One-foot bounce while bending other knee, with lower leg pointing back.

1 count

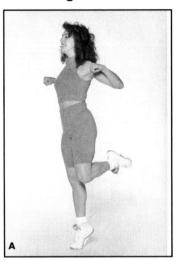

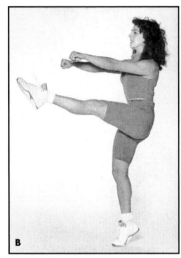

One-foot bounce and kick same leg forward, waist-high or lower.

1 count

Figure 7.12. Bounce 'n Tap Series

One-foot bounce on left (L) foot, pointing and tapping R toe forward. Arms punch parallel forward.

1–4 counts

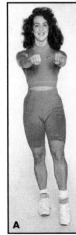

Weight remains on L bouncing, R toe now pointing and tapping wide R. Arms follow, wide to sides, palms/fists up.

1–4 counts

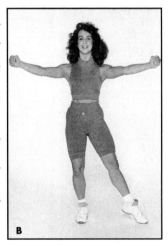

Weight remains on L bouncing, R toe now pointing and tapping backward. Arms raise overhead, thumbs back.

1–4 counts

Next: Alternate by bringing pointing and tapping foot in, and two-foot bounce in place.

1–4 counts

Shift weight to R foot and repeat series.

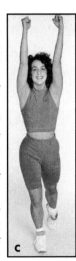

■ LOW-IMPACT AEROBICS

Figure 7.13. Heel-Toe Bounce Series

Bounce R foot while L heel extends forward. Arms forward.

1 count

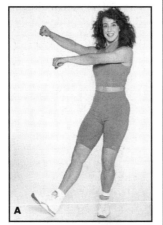

A

Bounce R foot, while L toe now taps in close. Draw arms in to chest.

1 count

Repeat heel out, followed by feet back in together in a transitional move.

1 count

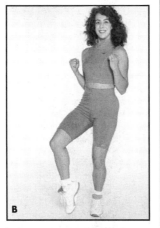

B

Figure 7.14. Kicks

Weight on one foot, kick other leg to only a **90° waist-high level** (or lower). Forward or sideward.

1 count

Bounce added.

2 counts

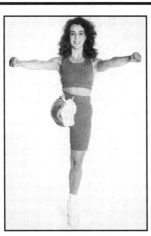

Figure 7.15. Knee-Lift Varieties

Step R, knee-lift L knee forward, same elbow touch.

2 counts

Reverse.

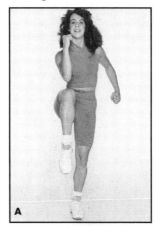

A

Step R, knee-lift L knee sideward, same elbow out wide and touch.

2 counts

Reverse.

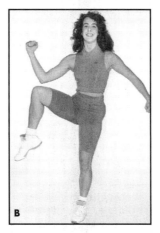

B

Step R, knee-lift L knee across body center forward, R (i.e., opposite) elbow across chest and touching the knee-lifted.

2 counts

Reverse.

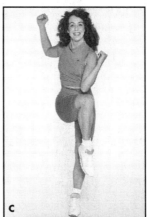

C

■ LOW-IMPACT AEROBICS

Figure 7.16. Lunge Side and Bounce

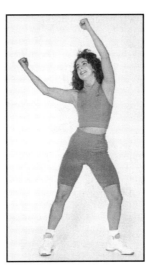

Step and bounce-lunge R, arms overhead, parallel, and diagonally high L, head following direction of arms.

2 counts

Reverse, shifting weight.

2 counts

Figure 7.17. Marching

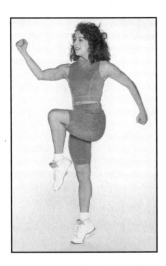

Step-lift, one count each step pattern. Arms swing opposite and **big**.

1 count

Figure 7.18. Side Step-Out

Step out wide stride to R side, bending knees.

1 count

Clap hands R.

1 count

Reverse.

2 counts

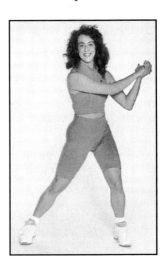

Note Low-impact aerobics are any exercise-dance movements in which one foot always has contact with the floor and that fulfill the other aerobic criteria established in Chapter 2.

■ POWER LOW-IMPACT WITH PLYOMETRIC MOVES

[Figures 2.9; 4.5–4.6] 7.19–7.21[2]

Figure 7.19. Two-Foot Jump

Step 1

Lift high on balls of feet, without leaving floor.

1 count

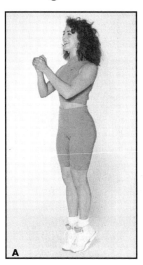

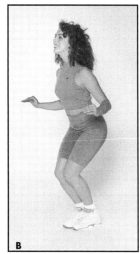

Step 2

Land and gently **press the heels** into the floor.

1 count

Figure 7.20. Knee Lift

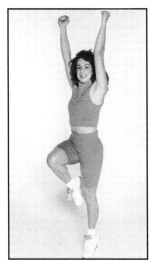

Lift knee while rising to **ball** of foot.

1 count

Be sure to lower heel of support foot as lifted foot returns to floor.

1 count

Arms forcefully assist in **raising** entire body, reaching above shoulder level.

Figure 7.21. Twist

Shift weight from ball of foot, to ball of foot, as you lift your body and twist from side to side.

2 counts

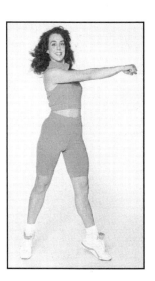

Note　You can easily use these moves as moderate-impact plyometric moves — lunges [Figure 2.6-2.8], jumps, kicks, step-touches, jogs, heel-jacks, ponies.[3]

■ HIGH-IMPACT AEROBICS

Figures [4.7] 7.22–7.33

With high-impact locomotor (movements that take you from place to place through space) activities, you are briefly airborne and have **a take-off** and **a landing**. The five basic high-impact locomotor movements are the following:[4]

Take-Off	Landing	Example	Figure
One foot	same foot	hop; hitch-kick	7.22–7.23
One foot	opposite foot	leap; rock	7.24; 7.25–7.26
One foot	two feet	astride	7.27
Two feet	two feet	jump (together or wide-stride)	7.28–7.29
Two feet	one foot	hopscotch	7.30

The following illustrate the five basic take-offs and landings found in high-impact aerobics. Limit repetitions of the same impact landing to **four or fewer** to avoid overuse and injury.

Figure 7.22. Hops – Single and Double

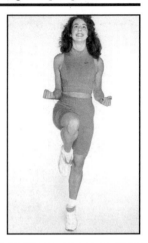

Single Hops:
Hop R, forward lifting L knee.

1 count

Double Hops:
Repeat R hop.

2 counts

Figure 7.23. Hitch-Kick

Step 1

Hop on L as R foot lifts back, knee bent.

Option:
Arms forcefully pulling back.

1 count

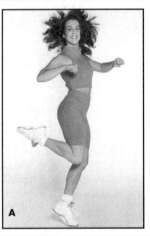

A

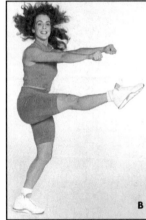

B

Step 2

Hop L again, kicking R forward, waist-high or lower.

Option:
Arms forcefully parallel punching forward.

1 count

Reverse.

2 counts

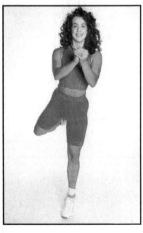

Figure 7.24. Leap

With weight L (not shown) take-off, propelling body forward and upward, landing on R foot.

4 counts

Figure 7.25. Rock Side-To-Side

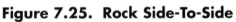
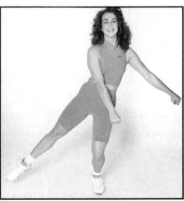

Hop on R foot to R side, placing weight over R leg (knee and ankle flexed), lifting L leg out to the side.

1 count

Reverse.

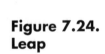

■ HIGH-IMPACT AEROBICS

Figure 7.26. Rock Forward

Rock (hop) R into a forward lean, lifting L leg back and up for balance.

1 count

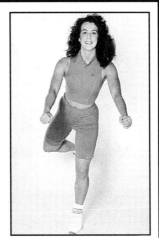

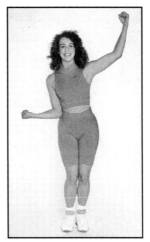

Figure 7.29. Jumps – Feet Together

Jump sideward, forward, or back. Hold.

2 counts

Reverse.

Option: Use skiing arms position with L elbow **close**, R elbow high and wide, when jumping R. Reverse arms when you reverse feet.

Note   When executing two-foot jump to the side in wide-stride position, followed by two-foot jump together, this becomes a Jumping Jack (see 4.7). Arms can work wide and together with legs, or in opposition.

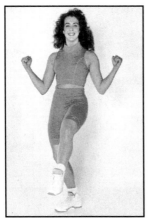

Figure 7.27. Rock Backward

Rock (hop) L backward into a backward lean, lifting R leg forward and up for balance.

1 count

Figure 7.30. Lunge or Wide-Stride

Two-foot scissors jump forward on R foot, bending R knee as L leg is kept extended back (still bearing weight on L) in wide forward/ backward lunge position. L arm forward, R arm back.

1 count

Options: (1) Jump back to **two-feet together** and center, **1 count**, then reverse the forward and backward legs and arms lunging and jumping back to center.

2 counts.

(2) Reverse **directly** from forward/back-ward lunge, (**1 count**) to opposite forward/backward lunge position.

1 count

Figure 7.28. Stride

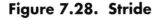

Weight R or L (not shown) hop to astride or straddle position, loading weight onto both feet by bending knees.

1 count

(Usually preceded by or followed with another move.)

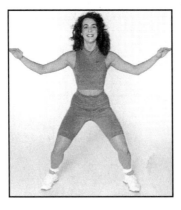

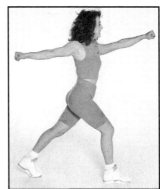

■ HIGH-IMPACT AEROBICS

Figure 7.31. Hopscotch – Back

Hop to stride position (not shown), and with weight on L foot, hop and touch R foot raised **backward** to lowered L hand.

2 counts

For balance, reach R hand diagonally skyward, thumb **back**. Reverse.

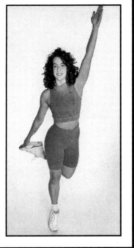

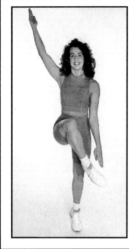

Figure 7.32. Hopscotch – Forward

Hop to stride position (not shown) and with weight on R foot, hop and touch L foot raised forward to lowered R hand (a knee open position). 2 counts.
For balance, reach L hand diagonally skyward, thumb **back**. Reverse.
Note: If you have sensitive (injury-prone or recent surgery) knees, avoid this exercise variety.

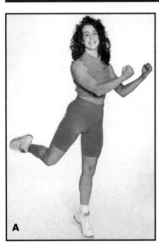

Figure 7.33. Polka

Many established popular social dances, or dance steps and gestures, are incorporated in the aerobics class setting.[5]

Hop R, lifting L leg backward.

1 count

Step L, in close quickly.

1/2 count

Step R, in close quickly.

1/2 count

Step L, in close quickly.

1/2 count

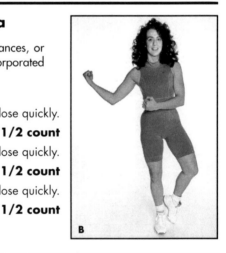

■ HIGH / LOW-IMPACT AEROBICS   Figures [4.7–4.8]

This section of the aerobics class setting was described in depth in Chapters 2 and 4, so techniques can be reviewed there. Most *high-impact* moves can be easily converted to *low-impact* moves simply by removing the five basic high-impact locomotor movements just detailed. Instead of a take-off and landing, those moves are changed to moves:

- in which one foot remains on the floor as the free foot uses floor and air space; or
- keeping both feet on the ground, incorporating the lifting and lowering plyometric principles from Chapter 2.

To change low-impact moves to high-impact, you simply replace the stationary-foot move and incorporate the high-impact locomotor moves of take-offs and landings (i.e., hops, hitch-kicks, leaps, rocks, hop astride, two-foot jumps, or hopscotch-type moves replace a low-impact "step" move).

■ AEROBICS VARIETY: FUNK MOVES   Figures 7.34–7.36

Funk aerobics are exercise moves developed from the culturally rich areas of jazz dance, ballet, street dance, gymnastics floor-exercise competition, and other rhythmical forms of aesthetic, emotionally expressive movement.

Funk aerobics include numerous expressive trunk, elbow and knee moves, funk walking (Figure 7.34) that mimics movie and television characters, and animation moves such as Roger Rabbit and funky chicken.

Creative expression and attitude prevail in funk exercise movement. Body gestures include the extremely big and wide-open positions (Figure 7.35), followed quickly by closed, tight, head gesture or hair-tossing moves (Figure 7.36).

You'll find the only limitation for funk aerobics movement lies in your own resources of experience and your individual creativity — which for all of us is absolutely unlimited!

Figure 7.34.
Funk Walking

Figure 7.35.
Open Position

Figure 7.36.
Closed Position

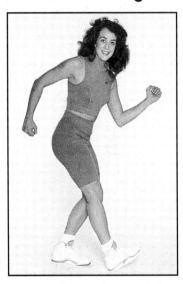
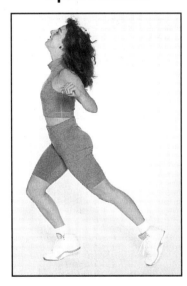
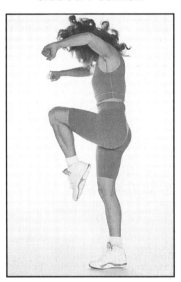

Summary of Aerobics Techniques

Low-impact, power low-impact, moderate-impact, high-impact, and "combo" have been described and detailed here so that you can design an individualized program according to your needs. Chapter 8 (Choreography) will assist you in designing a safe, challenging, and fun aerobics program. Table 8.1. is provided for you to develop an individualized program, incorporating your favorite impact moves, in combinations you choose.

The aerobic segment of your program can include many varieties: pace walking/jogging/ running, jumping rope, cycling, swimming, cross-country skiing, in-line skating, and the newest aerobics exercise modality that is taking the fitness industry by storm: step training and the use of light resistance while stepping.

Bench/Step Training Techniques

Figures 7.37–7.60

Techniques introducing the bench/step training with regard to bench height to choose, proper technique for stepping up and stepping down, and adding hand-held weights to increase intensity and further promote upper-body conditioning are described and shown in Chapter 5, Figures 5.1–5.5. Correct step training postures to avoid injuries are shown in Chapter 6, Figures 6.11–6.16.

The initial approach (step your first step of a pattern onto the bench), basic step movements, and how to add variety to the basic step movements and patterns are all presented here.

■ BENCH/STEP DIRECTION APPROACHES

Figures 7.37–7.42

If you're following the movements of an instructor, position the bench for maximum visibility. Initial movement onto the bench can begin from one of the following directions — **the direction in which your body faces the bench.**

Figure 7.37. From the Front

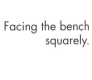
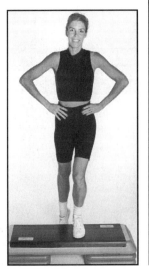

Facing the bench squarely.

Figure 7.38. From the End

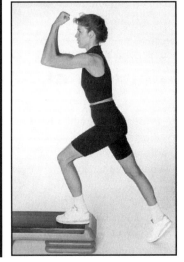

Facing the **end** of the bench, step up and down.

■ BENCH/STEP DIRECTION APPROACHES

Figure 7.39. From the Side

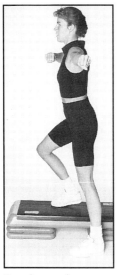
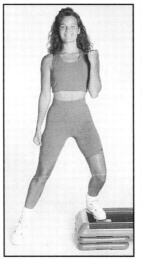

Standing with **your side** next to the bench's **side**, step up with the foot that is closest to the side of the bench.

Standing with **your side** next to the **end** of the bench, step up with the foot that is closest to the side of the bench.

Figure 7.41. From the Top

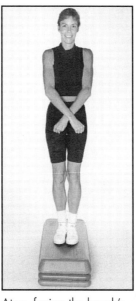
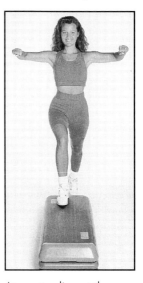

Atop, facing the bench's **end**, with feet together (shown); or feet in a forward/backward stride.

Atop, standing at the back end of the bench, step off the back in a forward/backward stride.

Figure 7.40. Astride/ Straddle

Facing the bench's **end**, standing astride or straddle position, with bench between your feet.

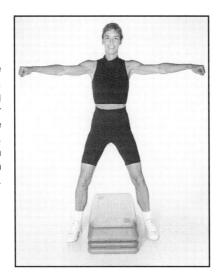

Figure 7.42. From the Diagonal

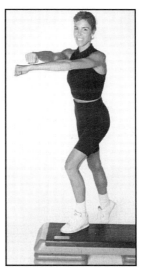

Facing on an angle toward corner when beginning a by-pass pattern (i.e., second move "by-passes" the bench and is a knee-lift, kick, etc.).

■ BASE STEPS

There are three base steps which may be performed using a variety of directional approaches/orientations. They are identified as:

- a **single** lead step, in which the **same** foot leads **every 4-count cycle**;
- an **alternate** lead step — the right and left foot both serve as the lead foot **alternately initiating every 4 counts**, requiring a complete cycle for the alternating patterns to **take 8 counts** (i.e., both the right foot and then left foot lead a 4-count portion of the cycle);
- a **step touch**, performed by "touching" the *same* toe or heel on the floor or bench (a 2-count move) or by *alternating* legs. Step touch moves are often used during the warm-up segment to familiarize you with the bench, or as transition moves during the aerobic segment.

For both safety and variety when using single-lead step, 4-count cycle patterns, lead with the right foot for a **maximum of 1 minute**, then change to a left-foot lead. To accomplish this change in lead foot (for single cycle 4-count step patterns), perform a **non-weight-bearing, transitional, hold/touch/tap/heel** move as the last step of the cycle, initiating the change with that foot.

> **Within the descriptions, only the moves typed in bold face are shown in the figures.**

Figure 7.43. Single Lead Step

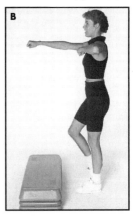

Bench Approach: Front (shown), top, end, and diagonal

	R	L	L	L	
Right Lead:	**Up**	up	down	**down**	**4 counts**

	L	R	L	R	
Left Lead:	Up	up	down	down	**4 counts**

Arms shown: Long-lever punching on up, up; pull, punch, on the down, down.

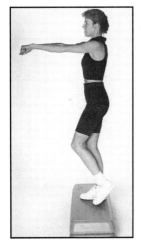

Alternating Lead Step

You can alternate the lead leg with a bench tap up (on bench) or a floor tap down (on floor).

Bench approach: Front (shown), top, end, and diagonal.

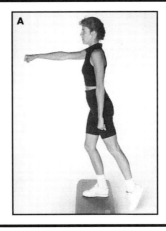

Figure 7.44. Bench Tap

R	L	L	R
Up	**bench tap**	down	down

Alternate (i.e. Up (L), bench-tap (R), down (R), down (L). **8 counts**

Arms shown: Forward punching.

Figure 7.45. Floor Tap

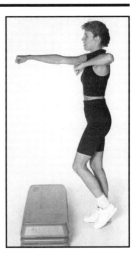

R	L	R	L
Up	up	down	**floor tap**

Alternate.   **8 counts**

Arms shown: Opposite arm long-lever punching; same arm flexing, elbow kept shoulder high.

■ BASE STEPS

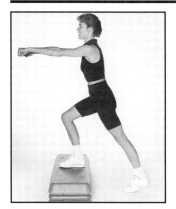
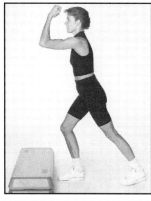

Figure 7.46. Lunge Back

Note: The Floor Tap can also be a non-weight-bearing lunge back.

R	L	R		L
Up	up	down	**down and back**	

Alternate.   **8 counts**.

Arms shown: Arms punching forward and parallel on up, up; bicep curls keeping elbows still high on the down, down.

Figure 7.47. Step Touch

Bench Approach: Front (shown), top, end, astride

        R   R
Bench-tap with toe   down;   repeat with left foot.

4 counts

Arms shown: Elbows shoulder-high, fists together on tap; fists apart on down.

Option: Try a Bench Tap using the **heel**, instead of the toe.

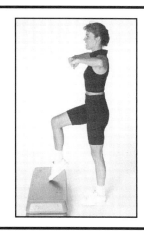

■ BASIC STEP PATTERNS[6]

Figures 7.48–7.54

Basic step patterns may be performed as single lead steps (4-count pattern) or alternating lead steps (8-count pattern). When performing a **single lead basic step pattern**, the **fourth count** of the cycle is weight-bearing. When executing **alternating lead steps**, there are two options — when the first 3 steps are weight-bearing the 4th is **non-weight bearing** or when the first 3 steps contain a bypass move, the 4th step is **weight-bearing**.

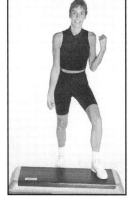
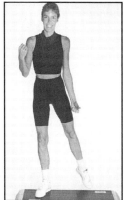

Figure 7.48. V-Step

Bench Approach: Front.

R	L	R	L
Up-wide	up-wide	**down-center**	down-center

Usually cued: "out" "out" "in" "in".

Arms shown: Same-side single bicep curls.

■ BASIC STEP PATTERNS – Bypass Bench Variations   Figures 7.49–7.52

Bench Approach: Front (shown), side, top, end, diagonal

Figure 7.49. Knee up Bypass[7]

L   R
Up,   **knee lift**   (bypasses the bench and lifts)

     R   L
down (to floor)   down (to floor).

Arms shown: Initiate from arms fully extended out to the sides shoulder high with palms up: Single short-lever curls on the up and knee lift; return one at a time to the long-lever, shoulder-high initial position on the down, down.

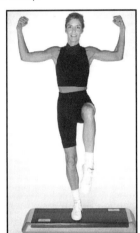

Figure 7.51. Kick Forward Bypass

L   R   R   L
Up **kick forward** down (to floor) down (to floor).

Arms shown: Arms sweep up from sides, together and parallel on up, kick; sweep together and parallel back down to sides on the down, down.

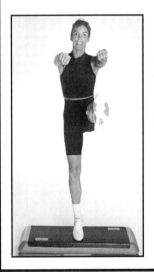

Figure 7.50. Kick Back Bypass

L   R
Up   **kick back**   (a "**long lever** raising" motion)

     R   L
down (to floor)   down (to floor)

Arms shown: Initiate from arms fully extended down at sides: Raise same (one) elbow out wide to shoulder high with fist ending at waist, for the up and kick back; lower to initial position at side with each down, down.

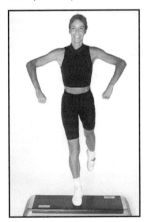

Figure 7.52. Side Leg Lift Bypass

L   R
Up **Side leg lift** (a knee pointing forward position),

     R   L
down (to floor)   down (to floor)

Arms shown: Both arms raised simultaneously to bent-arm lateral raise position for up; same arm (one) extends out to side shoulder high for the side leg lift; extended arm returns to bent-arm lateral raise on the down; both arms lowered simultaneously on the last down.

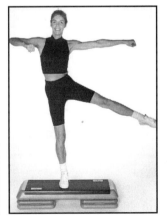

■ BASIC STEP PATTERNS

Figure 7.53. Straddle Down

Bench Approach: Top (shown).

R

Straddle Down (on R side of bench)

L

Straddle down (on L side of bench)

R   L
Up   Up

Arms shown: Shoulder high, short-levers, and fists together at center. Same long-lever arm extends out to side as same leg steps out. One arm at a time returns back in to center on each up, up step.

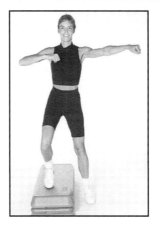
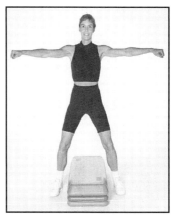

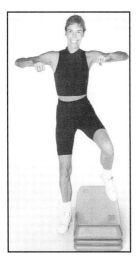
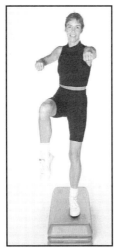

Figure 7.54. Straddle Up

Bench Approach: Astride (shown).

R   L
Up   **knee lift** (bypasses bench and lifts waist-high),

L   R
straddle down (to floor)   straddle down (to floor).

Arms shown: Same initial position as last pattern, with opposite arm punching forward on lift.

Note: For variety, try the other bypass moves shown earlier — kick forward, kick back, or side leg lift, incorporating one or more accompanying arm movements that will keep your balance atop the bench.

■ VARIATIONS OF BASE STEPS & BASIC STEP PATTERNS

Figures 7.55–7.60

To add variety to base steps and basic step patterns, a number of variations can be implemented. Several are shown here and categorized as traveling, repeaters, or propulsions. Creative arm movements will also play a significant role in adding variety and interest to the step training workout.

■ VARIATIONS – Traveling Patterns

Figures 7.55–7.56

Figure 7.55. Turn Step — Length of the Bench

Bench Approach: Side (shown).

Single lead – 4 counts; Alternating lead – 8 counts.

L	R	L	R
Up	**body 1/2 turns left and up**	**down**	**tap-down**

Arms shown: Shoulder-high alternating punch and pull back.

> **Note** Remember to keep your eyes on the platform. Also, this pattern is shown using natural photography and descriptive words, since it could not be photographed, and therefore described, from a "mirrored" perspective.

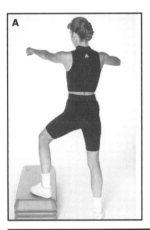 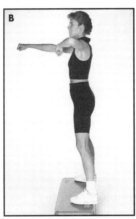 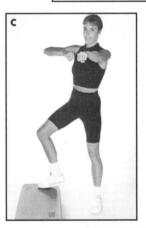 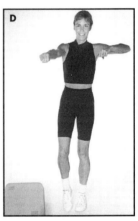

Figure 7.56. Over the Top — Width of the Bench

Bench Approach: Side (shown).

Single lead – 4 counts; Alternating lead – 8 counts.

L	R		
		L	R
Up	**up**	**down on the left side of bench/platform**	**touch-down**

Alternate. Cued: "up", "over", "down", "tap".

> **Note:** For variety on the *fourth* step, instead of tapping the floor, touch heel on bench; knee up; or kick front.

Arms shown: Elbows pointing skyward and shoulder high, with arms wide open on the first, third, fifth, and seventh steps; arms low and crossed in front on even-numbered steps.

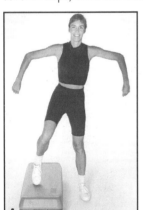 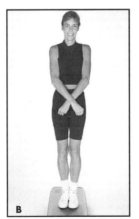 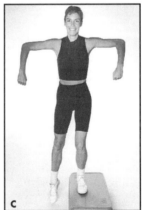 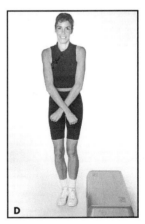

■ VARIATIONS OF BASE STEPS & BASIC STEP PATTERNS[8]

Figure 7.57. Repeaters

These are repetitions of any **non-weight-bearing move** and can be a single or alternating lead step. Keep the number of repeaters limited to a maximum of 4.

For example: Using a diagonal front approach, **step up**, **tap up**, **tap down and back**, tap up, tap down and back, tap up, step down (R), step down (L) squarely facing the front of the bench.

For variety, instead of taps use knee-lifts, forward kicks, kick-backs, side leg-lifts, etc.

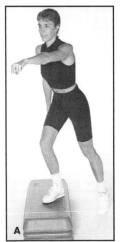
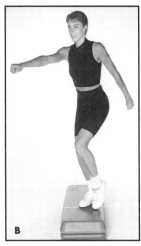
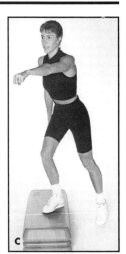

Figure 7.58. From the End

You create an 8- or 16-count step pattern that utilizes **all three sides** of the bench, beginning from the end of the bench. When you get creative, **do not ever have your back facing the bench** while stepping up. Only three sides of the bench are available to you for any one pattern.

Steps **from the end** use multiple bench-approaches and multiple basic step patterns. Try the sample pattern diagrammed in Figure 7.58, and then continue creating your own patterns on page 114.

The figure illustrates an empty bench with sequential placement location of each foot. Beginning from the bench's end and with your weight on your **right foot** on the floor, step up on bench to the #1 location with your **left** foot. Continue on with the pattern, placing your next foot atop/on the side/or at the end — on the floor, wherever the sequential number indicates for foot placement.

Note   When alternating the pattern, final step 16 is a step (taking weight onto L foot). The next move is up (R). And, when changing to creating a totally new

pattern, final step #16 is a non-weight bearing move (like a "tap"), with the next weight-bearing step on that same ("tap") foot, either in place on the floor, or up, on the bench.

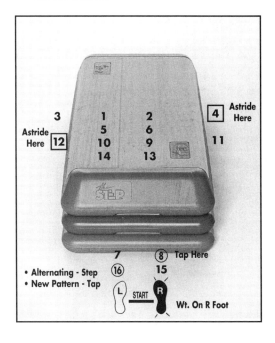

■ INTERMEDIATE/ADVANCED VARIATIONS[9]   Figures 7.59–7.60

During high-impact step patterns, (i.e., you are airborne during a portion of the pattern), hand-held weights are not used for safety reasons.

Figure 7.59. Propulsion Steps

Both feet push off the ground or bench, exchanging positions during the airborne phase of the pattern. Propulsion steps are commonly used with touch and lunge steps.[10] **4 counts.** Propulsion moves can also be used when performing bypass or traveling moves by adding a hop, or pushing off the foot on the bench.

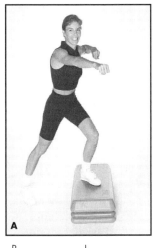

R   L
Up **lunge down and back**

2 counts

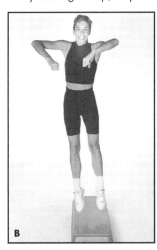

R
Push off   (with propulsion into this **airborne position**).

1 count

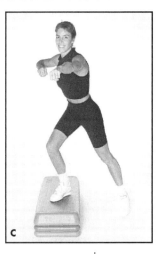

L
Landing on the opposite foot up, and the other foot (R) **lunging down and back**.

1 count

Figure 7.60. Adding Hand-Held Weights To Step Training[11]

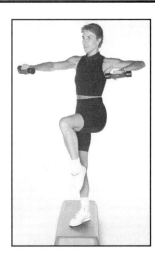

Extensive criteria for using hand-held weights are given in Chapter 5. *Once you are proficient at stepping,* adding 1-4 lb. hand-held weights can add intensity and variety to your program. The key to adding hand-held weights to step training is maintaining excellent body positioning throughout and being in absolute control of the weights for all upper body movement gestures. Firm "strength/weight training"-type arm movements such as long-lever raises and short-lever curls, symmetrical or in combination as shown in Figure 7.60, are the type of arm movements used for stepping, rather than the more fluid, free-flowing gestures sometimes used in aerobics.

Bench/Step Training Techniques Summary

Techniques illustrating the fundamentals of step training presented here include:

- Methods to directionally approach the bench.
- The three base steps.
- The basic step patterns.
- Variations of base steps and basic step patterns.

As you advance in your fitness and stepping skills, adding variety will become your next challenge, not only by developing more intricate foot patterns but also by adding many powerful arm movements, taken primarily from strength-training principles. Chapter 8, detailing the principles of choreography, will challenge your creative potential for putting unique possibilities together. Table 8.2 is provided for you to begin developing an individualized program, incorporating your favorite step training moves, in the combinations you choose.

Potential and possibilities for using the step-bench do not stop with just aerobic step training. Its versatility can extend into all of the final or initial segments of your total fitness program hour. To encourage your exploring this versatile, yet inexpensive, piece of equipment in conjunction with the final segments of your aerobics class workout, the exercise techniques presented for the final two program segments will center on using this exciting new equipment.

> **Note:** Directly preceding the strength-training segment or stretching and relaxation that comes next will be several minutes of transitional cool-down movement. This serves primarily to slow down the pulse, breathing, and other physiologies that have been working quite intensely. You can accomplish this transition with the step-bench by performing a variety of big arm gestures with slow, bench-tapping, step touch types of moves.

3. STRENGTH-TRAINING

The strength training segment is optional in the aerobics class setting but, as it is a vital component of your total physical well-being, most aerobics classes today include 10–20 minutes of strength-training to provide a well-balanced and complete fitness program. Guidelines from the American College of Sports Medicine state that "strength training of a moderate intensity, sufficient to develop and maintain fat-free weight, should be an integral part of an adult fitness program. One set of eight to twelve repetitions, of eight to ten exercises that condition the major muscle groups, at least two days per week, is the recommended minimum."[12] Thus, the prescription for more fully developing your lean (fat-free) weight is:

Set	Reps	Varieties of Exercises	Minimum Days/Week
1	8–12	8–10	2
		targeting major muscle groups	(with max.: 4/week, or every other day)

You can continue to enjoy using the step bench for the strength-training segment, focusing on the following isolated muscle groups of the upper, mid, and lower body.

- Upper body: chest, upper back, shoulders, and arms.
- Mid section: abdominals, lower back.
- Lower body: hips and buttocks, thighs, and lower legs.

Techniques presented here use the following types of weight resistance modes:

- Commercial rubber resistance bands.
- Commercial rubber resistance tubing alone, or with the aid of the bench.
- Gravity-assisted techniques, in which the bench is placed in an incline or decline position, with 1–4 pound* hand-held weights, resistance tubing, or using your own body weight as the sole resistance.

The exercises illustrated and described here have been categorized according to the location of the muscle group(s) benefited (upper body/mid section/lower body) using a variety of equipment. Be sure to breathe evenly on all strength-training exercises. It's never acceptable to hold your breath and turn red. Your working muscles constantly need oxygen. Figure 7.61 illustrates the major muscle groups to be strength-trained, and Table 7.1 identifies the exercises that will accomplish the training.

---

* The bench is not designed for using free-weights that weigh more than 10 pounds.[13] For comfort and safety, place a towel on the bench platform when lying on it.

MUSCLE STRUCTURE

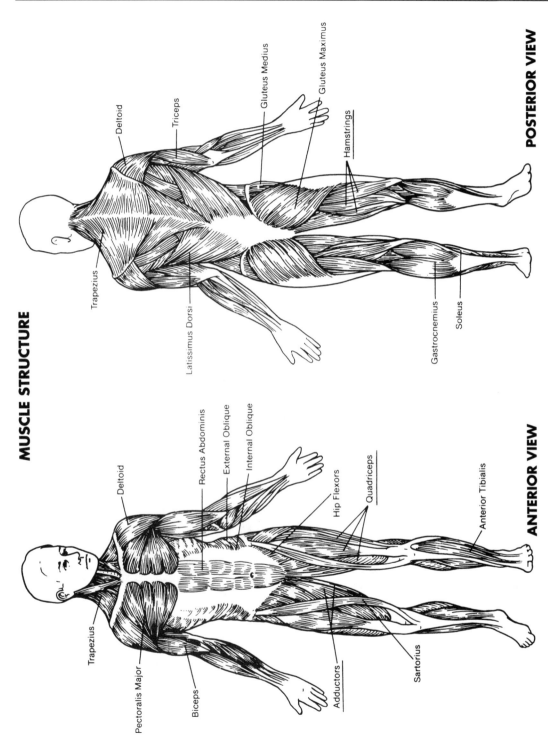

POSTERIOR VIEW

Redrawn from F. D. Giddings, 1980

ANTERIOR VIEW

FIGURE 7.61. The major muscles to be strength-trained.

From James L. Hesson, *Weight Training for Life* (Englewood, CO: Morton Publishing, 1985, pp. 164–165.

Figures [4.14–4.21; 4.23–4.27] 7.62–7.84

TABLE 7.1. Strength Training Exercises Using Various Forms of Resistance[14,15,16]

UPPER BODY Chest/Upper Back/Shoulders/Arms	MID-SECTION Abdominals/Low Back	LOWER BODY Hips and Buttocks/Thighs/Lower Legs
▪ Chest (Pec) Cross-Over ▪ Bent-Arm Chest Cross-Over ▪ Seated Lat Row ▪ Lat Pull Down ▪ Deltoid Lateral Raise (band/tubing) ▪ Deltoid Lateral Raise with Squat ▪ Upright Row ▪ Bicep Curl (tubing/band) ▪ Bicep Curl with Squat ▪ Tricep Kick (Press) Back (band/tubing) ▪ Overhead Press	▪ Gravity-Assisted Curl-Up with Weights ▪ Reverse Curl-Up ▪ Back Extension	▪ Buttocks/Heel Lift ▪ Side Leg Raise ▪ Inner Thigh Lift ▪ Leg Curl ▪ Heel Raise with Squat ▪ Seated Lower Leg Flexor and Extensor

■ UPPER BODY — CHEST • UPPER BACK • SHOULDERS • ARMS

Figure 7.62. Chest (Pec) Cross-Over

Tubing　　　　　　　　　　　　(Pectorals)

Position: Step on tubing with one or both feet, with slight bend in knees. Arms are away from body, in front of thighs, no tension.

Action: Cross arms at midline, wrists locked, elbows bent.

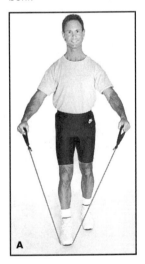
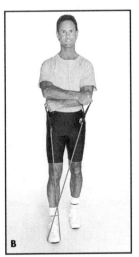

Figure 7.63. Bent-Arm Chest Cross-Over

Bench and Tubing　　　　　　　　(Pectorals)

Position: Sit center, move buttocks to lower third of bench, lie with head resting at top. Grab tube under platform at top block where it is grooved. Feet flat on floor, knees in open position.

Action: Cross-punch arm position over chest.

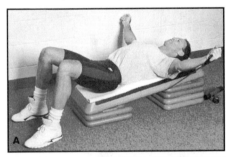
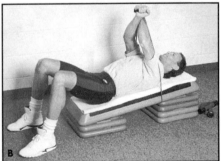

■ UPPER BODY — CHEST • UPPER BACK • SHOULDERS • ARMS

Figure 7.64. Seated Lat Row   Tubing   (Lats/Trapezius/Rear Deltoid)

Position: Seated, with both knees bent, toes pointed forward, abdominals contracted (to protect lower back). Hands at waist level, fists facing, arms away from body.

Action: Pull elbows behind body, fists facing sides; keep head and spine stationary.

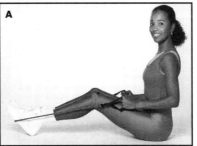
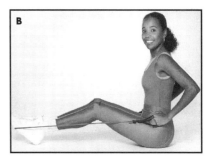

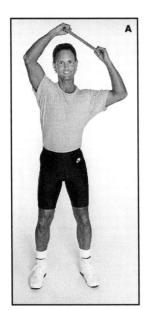
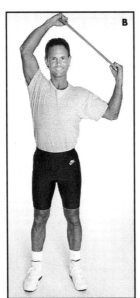

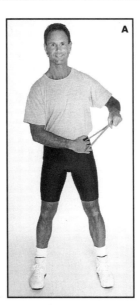
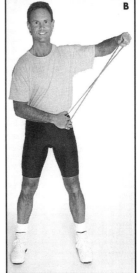

Figure 7.65. Lat Pull Down

Band   (Latissimus Dorsi)

Position: Grasp band with L hand and place overhead. L elbow is slightly bent, and band is anchored above/behind center of your head.

Action: Grasp band with R hand, keeping hand away from R ear, slowly pull down so R elbow comes into R side of body. Control the return.

Figure 7.66. Deltoid Lateral Raise

Band   (Deltoids/Trapezius)

Position: Grasp band with L hand and anchor it on R hip/side/thigh. Grasp band with R hand, firm fist facing side, elbow bent.

Action: Pull slowly out wide to shoulder height.

■ UPPER BODY — CHEST • UPPER BACK • SHOULDERS • ARMS

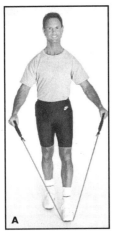 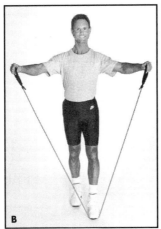

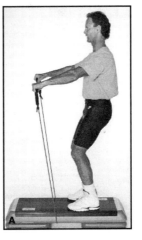 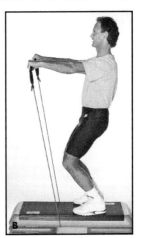

Figure 7.67. Deltoid Lateral Raise

Tubing   (Deltoids/Trapezius)

Position: Step on tubing with R foot while L foot is behind and L of midline, knees and elbows slightly bent.

Action: Raise elbows away from sides up to shoulder-level while keeping wrists/forearms locked, and hands slightly higher than elbows.

Figure 7.68.
Deltoid Lateral Raise with Squat

Bench and Tubing   (Deltoids/Trapezius)

Position: Stand on top of bench with tubing under center, having a fists top/thumbs in and down position.

Action: Press up, bending knees, with hands leading, going only to shoulder level or lower. If fatigued, raise arms just half way.

Figure 7.69. Upright Row

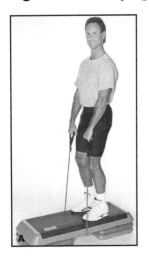 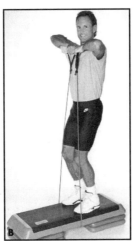

Bench and Tubing   (Deltoids/Trapezius)

Position: Initial foot and tubing position are the same, hands/fists now facing and resting on thighs.

Action: Raise handles up to chin, flaring out elbows slightly, keeping spine firmly erect.

> **Note** Bent knees in all of these illustrations assist in keeping a target heart rate, so that these exercises also can serve as 1 minute strength-training "intervals" in aerobic step-training with strength programs.

■ BICEP CURLS

Figure 7.70. Bicep Curl

Tubing　　　　　　　　　　(Biceps/Brachialis)

Position: Step on tubing with one/two feet, slight bend in knees, and fists/palms facing body, wrists locked, elbows kept at sides throughout.

Action: Curl both arms toward shoulders.

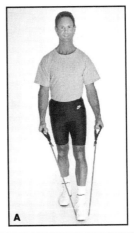
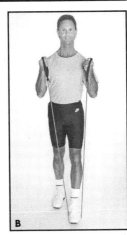

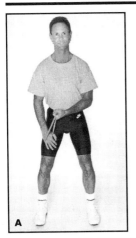
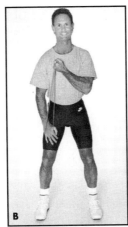

Figure 7.71. Bicep Curl

Band　　　　　　　　　　　　(Biceps)

Position: L hand anchors band on L thigh. Grasp band with R hand, keeping wrist locked, and R elbow against side.

Action: Curl up arm past chest, wrist ending center and toward R shoulder.

Figure 7.72. Bicep Curl with Squat

Bench and Tubing　　　　(Bicep/Brachialis)

Position: Same standing, tube location as in Upright Row, and hand/fist position facing thighs.

Action: Curl up to sky, rotating palms on the way up so they face shoulders. Reverse rotation for return. Bend knees to increase heart rate.

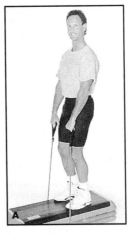
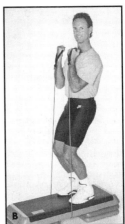

■ TRICEPS

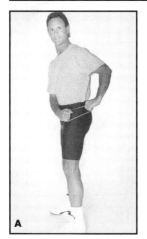
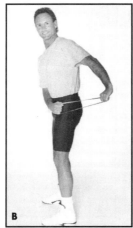

Figure 7.73.
Tricep Kick (Press) Back

Band   (Triceps)

Position: Grasp band with L hand and anchor it on R thigh. Grasp band with R hand, palm/fist facing backward, relaxed position. L arm bent and stabilized against body.

Action: Press arm back to fully extended position. Maintain good body position.

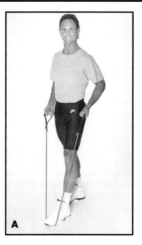
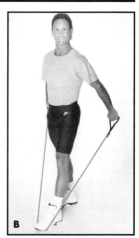

Figure 7.74.
Tricep Kick (Press) Back

Tubing   (Triceps)

Position: Stand in forward/back stride position, grasp handles with palms facing up/in, elbows cocked.

Action: Press both arms backward, rotating wrists so palms are facing rear, firm wrists, arms fully extended.

Figure 7.75. Overhead Press

Incline Bench and Tubing   (Deltoids/Triceps)

Adjust bench so two blocks are at low end and four blocks are at high end.

Position: Prone, with tubing in back of second block's groove, hands starting at sides, wide, and chin resting on incline bench top.

Action: Press up and forward, ending with thumbs in and facing each other.

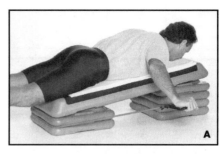

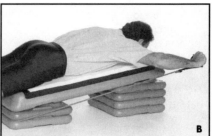

■ MID-SECTION — ABDOMINALS ■ LOW BACK

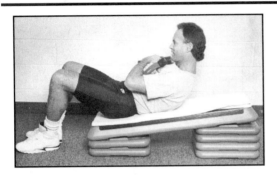

Figure 7.76.
Gravity-Assisted Curl-Up

Incline Bench and 1–4 lb. weights   (Abdominals)

Position: With bench in incline position, straddle and sit on lower third. Place 1–4 pound free-weights* on sternum (breastbone), with knees flared out wide and heels together, flat on floor.

Action: Keeping lower back on bench at all times, curl up, head looking forward. This is all the farther you go; release and curl back down to lying position.

*Adding more weight resistance is optional, but if you do, this is where it should be done. Maximum hand weights to use on bench is 10 lbs.

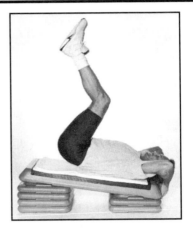

Figure 7.77. Reverse Curl-Up

Decline Bench   (Abdominals)

Position: Place bench in a decline position, lie on bench, face up with head at lower end of bench. Grasp lip of platform and top block over your head. Legs are skyward, with hips, knees, and ankles bent softly.

Action: Contract abdominals and raise buttocks up, keeping lower back on the platform. Lower.

Reps for abdominal work can be 15–30, and two sets — one before an aerobics session and one after — because the type of muscle tissue located here responds better to more repetitions for "definition" than other groups of the body do. These exercises are to help strengthen sensitive lower backs; the low back is completely supported during the abdominal contraction.

Figure 7.78. Back Extension

Incline Bench   (Erector Spinae)

Position: Lie prone with hips on lower third, legs extending off bench, supported by toes on floor. With chin on bench, place hands at hips area.

Action: Contract low back and raise upper chest; hands may move in a sliding motion backward. Lower.

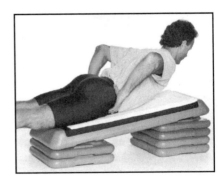

■ LOWER BODY — HIPS AND BUTTOCKS ■ THIGHS ■ LOWER LEGS

Figure 7.79. Buttocks/Heel Lift

Band   (Gluteals)

Position: Assume an all-fours position, resting on forearms, knees wider than hips, abdominals tight. Place band around L ankle and R instep.

Action: Bend R leg with heel pointing to ceiling, lifting heel without bending knee any further, going as far as band will allow. Lower. Alternate legs to achieve balance.

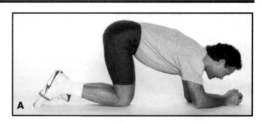

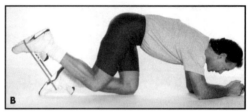

Figure 7.80. Side Leg Raise

Band   (Thigh Abductors)

Position: Place band just above knees. Lie on side, with head resting on bottom arm which is straight overhead. Top arm is in a bent-arm support in front of chest, with legs either slightly bent or knees bent to 90 degrees.

Action: Raise top leg (bent as shown) 6–12 inches, toward ceiling. Control body position during raising and lowering. After reps, change position and alternate, to strengthen both legs.

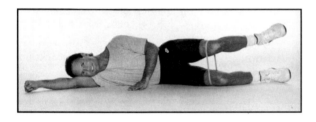

Figure 7.81. Inner Thigh Lift

Band   (Thigh Adductors)

Position: Lie on side with band placed around instep of both feet. Cross top leg forward, over bottom leg, and place foot flat on floor.

Action: Lift bottom leg up toward ceiling as far as you can, with toes slightly higher than heel. Lower leg slowly, not allowing it to touch floor. After reps are completed, alternate legs.

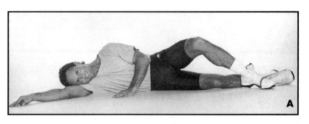

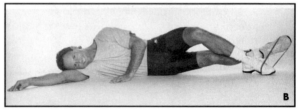

■ LOWER BODY — HIPS AND BUTTOCKS ■ THIGHS ■ LOWER LEGS

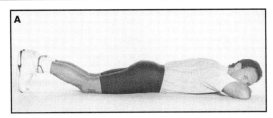

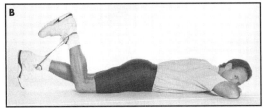

Figure 7.82. Leg Curl

Band   (Hamstrings)

Position: Lie face down, with band around ankles.

Action: Bend R leg, bringing heel toward and within 12–18 inches of buttocks, keeping hips firmly down on floor. Return. Alternate.

Note: An excellent exercise for the Quadriceps, as a balance to this exercise, is shown in Chapter 4, Figure 4.24. Hips again are held firmly on the floor, and the action is alternated after the reps, for balance.

Figure 7.83. Heel Raise with Squat

Bench and Tubing   (Gastrocnemius/Soleus)

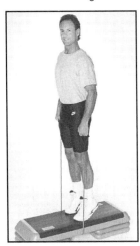

Position: Feet center, standing tall. Tubing is placed under center of bench, and held at sides of hips.

Action: Keeping palms stationary (they do not move) at sides, raise heels up, contracting calves ("squeeze"). Lower back down and bend knees. Maintain excellent body alignment.

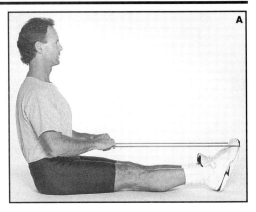

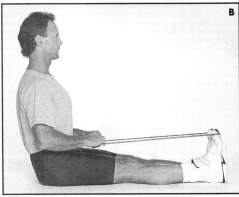

Figure 7.84. Seated Lower Leg Flexor and Extensor

Tubing   (Tibialis Anterior)

Position: Sit tall, chest raised, shoulders down, holding handles near thighs, palms down, with the tubing around the ball/toe area of both feet held close together.

Action: Without moving body or hands, point toes away from you.

Action: Now, without moving body or hands, point toes toward you, flexing ankles. This is a great exercise for prevention or relief of shin splints.

Strength Training Techniques Summary

This concludes an exciting variety of strength-training possibilities for you to try. Various equipment can be used to train the muscle groups, so whatever is your preference, or is available to you, you have at least one way to strength train each muscle group. (Even while you are traveling, you can easily pack the light resistance bands or tubing and continue your program uninterrupted.)

Recording your strength-training progress, choosing from this equipment, will prove to be a motivational blueprinting tool for you to continue with your program after the formal structure of an aerobics class setting ends. Record the following below and then continue in a journal:

- The specific exercise techniques you choose for your program.

- The number of sets and reps of each exercise you perform.

- The types of weight resistance used.

- The date of the workout.

Strength Training with Bands, Tubing, Light (1-4 lb) Free Weights & Tubing with the Bench							
Date							
Exercise	S / R / Res*	S / R / Res	S / R / Res	S / R / Res	S / R / Res	S / R / Res	S / R / Res
*S / R / Res = Sets, Repetitions, and Resistance (e.g., 3 / 8 / MT = 3 sets of 8 repetitions with medium tubing).							

4. COOL-DOWN, FLEXIBILITY TRAINING, AND RELAXATION

■ COOL-DOWN   Figures [4.28] 7.85

Figure 7.85.

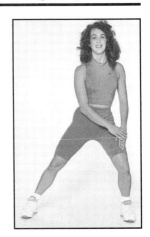

The purpose of a planned cool-down is to give your body time to readjust to the pre-activity state in which you began. According to whether you have just finished aerobics (exercise or step-training), or the optional strength training segment, the time may vary as to how long this transitional cool-down will require. Give yourself time to readjust your pulse, breathing, and other physiologies. Research tells us that the highest incidence of problems occur after an intense workout, so be sure to take this needed time (5 minutes minimum) to readjust. Movements are of a step-touch or wide-stride nature, with arms changing from big moves to decreasingly smaller moves.

■ FLEXIBILITY TRAINING
Figures [4.1–4.2; 4.11–4.13; 4.29–4.30; 7.3–7.10] 7.86–7.89

Stretching to increase your flexibility and range of motion is crucial now. It is a time when your muscles are warm (full of blood, oxygen, and nutrients) and your joints are pliable from vigorous exercise, so take full advantage of the next 5 to 10 minutes to static (or PNF) stretch. Many stretching techniques have been presented. Refer to any of them to incorporate into your flexibility training, or experiment on the step bench and try the following stretches.

Figure 7.86. Back Stretch

Sit on the end of the bench with your feet together on the floor. Bend over, resting your chest on thighs. Reach under legs with arms, grasp the opposite elbow and pull both elbows together. Hold.

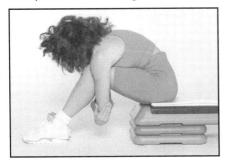

Figure 7.87. Pectoral Stretch

Lie down on the platform with head and buttocks both comfortably on bench. Press the low back into the bench and place arms out wide to the sides, shoulder level, and palms up. Relax arms as their weight falls toward the floor. Hold.

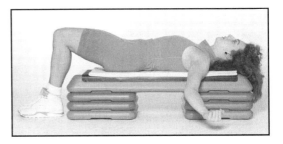

■ FLEXIBILITY TRAINING

Figure 7.88. Hamstring Stretch

Still lying on the bench, extend the L leg straight out along the platform, and place foot flat on floor. Grasp behind the R thigh and gently pull the R leg toward the chest. Hold.

Ankle Circling: During the hamstring stretch, slowly circle the foot in all directions. Alternate with L leg and foot.

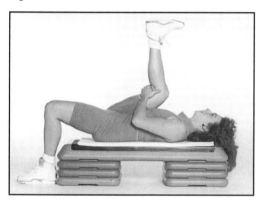

Figure 7.89. Achilles/Calf Stretch

From the hamstring stretch, pull R knee to chest. Grasp R toes with the hands and gently pull. Hold. Alternate with L leg and foot.

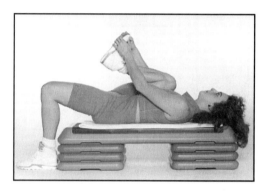

■ STATIC STRETCHING WITH RELAXATION   Figures [4.31] 7.90

At the conclusion of your workout hour, enjoy the natural high your beta endorphins are giving you, and begin relaxation techniques in the final stretching segment you perform. This is an excellent time to develop rich images and affirmations for yourself, starting with your energized muscles now becoming "wider-and-longer-and-warmer-and heavier." Your breathing is sequential with the pictures and affirmations. Breathe in deeply for 8 counts, hold the breath, and exhale and stretch (Figure 7.90) for 16 counts.

A complete program of relaxation techniques is presented in Chapter 9 to finalize your total physical fitness workout hour.

Figure 7.90.

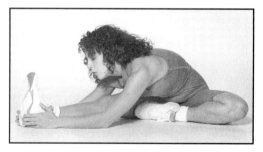

SUMMARY

This chapter has given you a basic blueprint of possible techniques to use for each of the four segments of an aerobics program. You'll next learn how to use these basic moves to create a lifetime of unlimited possibilities, as you try your skills at choreography!

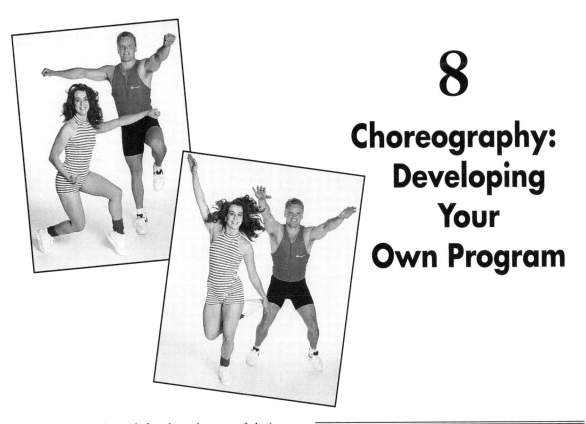

8

Choreography: Developing Your Own Program

Choreography is defined as the art of designing or planning movements.[1] Program development principles for choreographing aerobics and step-training can be metaphorically compared to the steps used to make a classic, time-honored recipe, which is actually just a plan or strategy. A time-honored recipe requires several consistent factors to achieve the same results that anyone can duplicate again and again. These are: the individual *ingredients* (key components), the *amounts* of each ingredient, and the *order* in which they are to be used.

Choreography likewise requires understanding of the key ingredients or basic components of a balanced program, the amounts, or movement possibilities and repetitions of those moves, and the order in which they are to be done (methodology). This constitutes the recipe or blueprint for choreography. The goal of this chapter is for you to become aware of these three consistent factors (*ingredients/amounts/order*) so you can become the creative source of your own personal program.

THE INGREDIENTS FOR BALANCED CHOREOGRAPHY

In both aerobics and step-training, exercise movements are planned around these three key ingredients:[2]

■ to satisfy the need for *biomechanical* safety — avoiding injury;

■ with *physiological* considerations in mind, to consistently achieve the overall training effect and other individual fitness goals you've set;

■ *psychologically*, to achieve both short-term, present-moment enjoyment and long-term satisfaction.

Freestyle choreography, or spontaneous improvisation workouts, are possible when you have advanced to the point at which all the elements of biomechanical safety, physiological intensity, and psychological pleasure have been permanently set in your mind and mastered (blueprinted). These principles then are intrinsic to your planning ability, expressed, moment-by-moment, as directed creative movement, coming spontaneously from your internal cueing resources.

PLANNING CONSIDERATIONS

Following are some of the main variables to consider when planning a well-balanced exercise program.

Floor Surface

For aerobics, wood floors are the first choice. Carpeted surfaces limit your lateral moves and eliminate all pivoting moves (for knee safety). Concrete surfaces have no *give* with impact. If concrete is the only floor surface available, use only low impact and non-locomotor (total body gesturing/no-impact) moves. For step-training, the floor surface should be non-skid, or the bench must have features that will keep it in place.

Fitness Level and Motor Skills of the Person(s)

Are you

- a novice to the activity?
- a beginner in fitness level or motor skills?
- an intermediate who is physically fit but has yet to master some of the basic motor skills involved?
- an intermediate with excellent motor skills who knows a lot of techniques but needs to become more physically fit?
- advanced in both physical fitness and motor skills?

Considerations here are the music tempo (speed) and how you cue and perform the movement (much slower for the novice and the beginner).

Gender and Former Movement Experience

Do you have athletic/strength training or a dance background? These considerations are especially important when planning the gestures to be used. The small distance between the wrist and the fingertips can make a difference. Men tend to prefer a fist or blade for most hand/palm gestures (Figure 8.1)[3] for both aerobics and step-training. Because this choreography is not performance-oriented but, rather, exercise-oriented, you may want to use only tension-filled hand/palm movements.

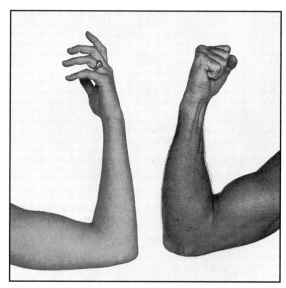

Figure 8.1. The small distance between the wrist and the fingertips can make a big difference in participation. Use exercise gestures that require tension-filled hands/palms.

Time-Frame

Knowing how much time you have will help to determine how long to make each of the various program segments. It may dictate whether you can add the fun and extra options, such as relaxation therapy.

Intensity of Moves

For aerobics, if you follow the instructions given earlier, you'll be able to keep the pulse safely in the training zone during the aerobic segment and lower during the warm-up, cool-down, strength-training, and stretching segments. The only additional requirement is that you have the skill of pulse-taking (and recognize RPE) and how to interpret the monitored pulse-reading, so you are responsible and accountable for your own program safety when it comes to heart rate intensity.

In addition, for step-training, recognizing when raising or lowering your intensity (by adding/subtracting hand-held weights, adjusting the bench height up or down, eliminating complex arm movements, or performing only on the floor or bench taps) is necessary.

Impact of Moves

Many times, simply using a wide variety of impacts with specific attention to repetitions of same-stress movements will do much to lessen negative stress upon the joints and the attending ligaments, tendons, and musculature. Also, shifting from mostly high-impact (airborne type) moves toward predominately low-impact and power low-impact moves (in which the impact is lessened because one foot is always grounded) is necessary to a safe, long-term program.

With the aforementioned points in mind, it becomes immediately apparent why the step-training phenomenon is sweeping the aerobics industry with unprecedented fervor! Providing a low-impact workout equal in musculoskeletal stress to a 3 mph pace walk and yet being able to experience the training effect benefits equal to a 7 mph run[4] obviously presents a terrific combination of safety and efficiency.

Kinesthetically Pleasing Moves

Kinesthetic, as defined in Chapter 1, means *internal bodily sensations*, encompassing three factors: emotions, muscle movements, and touch sense. Motor combinations should feel good. Moves that are intellectually challenging, yet easy to follow, keep your interest high.

AMOUNT = VARIETY AND REPETITIONS

When you decide to alter a recipe, you change several possibilities. You increase the same ingredients (such as the repetitions in choreography), or you carefully add new ingredients (variety of moves in choreography). Repetitions of moves have been adequately discussed. The remainder of this section lists the basics and then presents a variety of possibilities to add to those basics.

Movement Possibilities

Aerobics Impact Moves

These moves are described by the force exerted when the foot contacts the floor.

1. **Low-impact movement** (one foot always remains in contact with the floor):

- Bouncing Two-Feet
- Bounce'n Hitch-Kick
- Bounce'n Tap Series
- Half-Time Galloping
- Hoedown
- Heel-Toe Bounce Series
- Kicking (from ankle/knee/hip)
- Knee-Lift Varieties (forward/sideways/across)
- Lunging Varieties
- Marching
- Pace-Walking
- Side Step-Out
- Step-Touch

2. **Power low-impact movement** (forceful lifting and lowering):

- Heel Jacks
- Jogs
- Two-Foot Jumps
- Kicks
- Knee-Lifts
- Lunging
- Ponies
- Step-Touches
- Twist

3. **High-impact movement** (great force exerted when the foot contacts the floor; controlled landing is important):

- Jogging
- Jumping Varieties (single, stride, wide-stride or closed, hopscotch)
- Galloping
- Hopping Varieties (single, double, with kicks and knee-lifts)
- Hitch-Kick
- Leaping
- Polka
- Prancing
- Rocking
- Running
- Skipping
- Sliding

Step-Training Impact Patterns

In these patterns, one foot is always in contact with the bench or floor, or you are momentarily airborne.

1. **Low-impact basic step patterns** (one foot should always be in contact with the bench or floor):

- Single Lead Step
- Alternating Lead Step
  - Bench Tap
  - Floor Tap
  - Lunge Back
- Step Touch
- V-Step
- Straddle Down
- Straddle Up
- Bypass Bench Variations (knee up, kick forward, kick backward, side leg lift)
- Turn Step
- Over the Top
- Repeaters
- From the End

2. **High-impact variation** step pattern (momentarily airborne):

- Propulsion Steps

Gesturing

Gestures are movements of any non-weight-bearing body part (head, shoulders, fingers, hands, arms, torso, one leg, or foot).

1. **Basics:**

- Bending
- Circling
- Closing
- Curling
- Opening
- Pulling
- Pushing
- Shaking
- Stretching
- Swaying
- Swinging (arms/legs/torso)
- Tapping
- Turning
- Twisting

2. **Variations:**

- Different Style
  - Athletic-sports moves
  - Classic
  - Funk
  - Jazz
  - Martial arts
  - Military
  - Western
  - Create your own
- Adding Sounds
  - Claps
  - Finger Snaps
  - Slaps (thigh/ankles)
  - Specific gestures with audibles (military chants, shooting pistols, contact sounds, popular words and phrases)

Adding Variety to Basic Steps and Gestures

For both aerobics and step-training, the following applies to adding variety to your basic foot patterns and gestures.

1. **Vary the levers** (movement initiated from this joint):

- Arms:
  - From elbows — short lever moves
  - From shoulders — long lever moves
- Legs:
  - From knees — short lever moves
  - From hips — long lever moves

2. **Vary the planes and levels** (limbs move over and around the body):

■ Planes
  ■ Horizontal/vertical/diagonal

■ Levels
  ■ Low (knees), medium (chest), high (over-head)

3. **Vary the directionality and pathways** (movement toward/away from/or turning to face/an external directional point):

■ Directionality
  ■ Up/down
  ■ Right/left
  ■ Forward/backward
  ■ Diagonal

■ Pathways
  ■ Straight (lines/square/dueling sides)
  ■ Curved (spiral/double circle — same and opposite/two parallel ovals — partners meet and join)
  ■ Zig zag (V path/Z path)

4. **Vary the rhythm:**

■ How much movement or how many steps/gestures are performed in a unit of time (movement every beat; movement every other beat; movement at twice the tempo-speed of the beat)

■ Which beats are accented in a unit of time (*one*–2–3–4; 1–*two*–3–4; 1–2–*three*–4; 1–2–3–*four*; *one–two*–3–4; 1–2–*three–four*; *one and two*–3–4; 1–2–*three and four*; *one*– 2–*three*–4; 1–*two*–3–*four*; *one–two–three– four*)

5. **Vary the symmetry:**

■ Symmetrical movement (arms/legs/arms and legs/performing the same movement at the same time)

■ Asymmetrical movement (arms/legs/arms and legs/performing in opposition to one another)

6. **Vary the force** (of impacts and gestures):

■ According to:
  ■ Phase of the program
  ■ Current fitness levels
  ■ Motor skills

■ Range of possibilities:
  ■ No impact with low-intensity gestures
  ■ High-impact with high-intensity gestures

■ Under this category, should one use hand-held weights for aerobics programs? Criteria for safely using hand-held weights for aerobics are:

1. *Only* if you are at the *intermediate or advanced physical fitness* and motor skill level.

2, *Only* if you can maintain *a good body position* (posture) throughout the hour.

3. **Of key importance:** Only arm movements and gestures similar to those used for weight training (Figure 8.2) should be performed in aerobics when adding hand-held

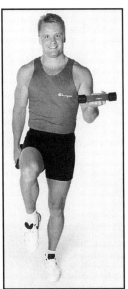 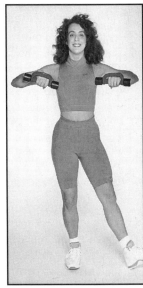

Figure 8.2. Knee lift with bicep curl.

Figure 8.3. Use only arm movements similar to those in weight training when adding hand-held weights.

weights (Figure 8.3). This means you must maintain absolute control of range of motion and velocity. Hand-held weights cannot be used safely for the fast, flailing movements characteristic of many aerobics programs. To safely add hand-held weights to the aerobic segment of your aerobics program, you must adapt considerably. The same three guidelines are appropriate for adding hand-held weights when step-training. More detailed guidelines for the use of hand-held weights during step-training are given in Chapter 5.

ORDER = METHODOLOGY

The movement possibilities presented in this chapter are put together in combinations called sequencing. The three variables around which the order of movement revolves are the three ingredients mentioned earlier: biomechanical safety needs, physiological intensity needs, and the psychological needs attendant to a positive, pleasant workout (intellectually challenging but easy to follow). Sequencing possibilities are:

1. **Continual progression of moves:** Performing isolated step/gesture movements. For example: an alphabet of moves such as

   (a) arm circles

   (b) bouncing and tapping

   (c) cross-step and hop.

2. **Add on:** Linking two moves together before adding another. You then can continually link, repeating all movement and adding on for a specific time frame. For example: sequence 1; sequence 1, add on 2; sequence 1, 2, add on 3.

3. **Pyramid:** Adding progressively more or fewer repetitions of moves or counts of music. For example: moves performed for 4–3–2–1 repetitions; or 1–2–3–4 repetitions. Many times, movement transitions execute well by adding a "hold" moves or count to the uneven-numbered repetitions, so the sequence fits smoothly into four or eight counts of music. The aerobics Bounce 'n Tap Series represents an excellent use of pyramid sequencing. It can be performed for an entire song, using either low-impact bouncing and directionally tapping, or high-impact hopping and tapping.

4. **Patterns:** Any two or more combinations of moves repeated in a certain repetitive cycle.

   ■ This is why the basics for step-training are usually described as patterns. Isolated steps can be part of the variety offered, but most of the movement is performed as two or more combinations of moves. Samples: Up, up, down, down; or up, kick, down, tap.

   ■ Many patterns together are present in a routine. Routines are start-to-finish choreographed movement.

SUMMARY

This chapter detailing choreography represents independence to you. It systematically delineates how movement is safely and efficiently planned to meet your needs. A two-sided worksheet entitled, "Creating Your Own Aerobics Routines" and "Creating Your Own Step Training Pattern Variations" has been developed for you to practice choreographing movement for an exercise session. Enjoy the unlimited aerobic movement possibilities when mixing and combining the variety of options offered here.

TABLE 8.1 Creating Your Own Aerobics Routines

IMPACT: AEROBIC MOVES:	LOW-IMPACT												HIGH-IMPACT															
	BOUNCING	■ 2 FT/HK/'N TAP	1/2 GALLOPING	HOEDOWN	HEEL-TOE	KICKS	KNEE-LIFTS	LUNGING	MARCHING	PACE-WALKING	SIDE STEP-OUT	STEP-TOUCHES	GALLOPING	HITCH-KICK	HOPPING	■ SINGLE/DOUBLE	■ W KICK	■ W KNEE-LIFT	JOGGING/RUN	JUMPING 2 FT.	■ STRIDE/CLOSED	■ HOPSCOTCH	LEAPING	POLKA	PRANCING	ROCKING	SKIPPING	SLIDING
GESTURE BASICS: ■ Bending - Twisting																												
GESTURE STYLE: ■ Athletic - Western																												
ADDED SOUNDS: ■ Claps/Snaps/Audible																												
LEVERS: ■ Arms Short/Long ■ Legs Short/Long																												
PLANES: ■ Horizontal/Vertical/ ■ Diagonal																												
LEVELS: ■ Low/Medium/High																												
DIRECTION: ■ Up/Down ■ Right/Left ■ Forward/Back ■ Diagonal																												
PATHWAY: ■ Straight ■ Curved ■ Zigzag																												
RHYTHM/BEAT ACCENTED: 1–2–3–4																												
SYMMETRY: ■ Symmetrical ■ Asymmetrical																												
FORCE OF: ■ Foot Impact ■ Gestures																												

TABLE 8.2
Creating Your Own Step Training Pattern Variations

Directions: Following all of the guideline given in Chapters 5 and 7, create your own patterns, From The End. Remember that for safety reasons only three sides of the bench can be used in a pattern. Start with a bench approach from the end, and proceed incorporating multiple basic step patterns and multiple bench approaches.

1. Indicate the location of the weight-bearing foot (WBF) to start the patterns, freeing the other foot to then be step #1. (The bench and floor has been divided into six sections for your convenience in placing the number locations.)

2. Begin the pattern by locating a "1" up on the bench (or down on the floor), followed with the location of the next step, identified as "2".

3. Continue on locating steps 3–8, then 9–16, identifying any step that has a key directive to be noted (i.e., ⑧ is a "tap" non-weight-bearing move; ⑫ you'll be in an astride position).

4. Identify any "bypass" step movement with a double circle around the non-weight-bearing foot location and labeling the type of bypass move, (i.e., ⑤ fwd. kick).

5. List arm gestures to accompany each step movement, plus any additional choreographed pointers (sounds, etc.) below, at right. Enjoy being creative!

STEPS:

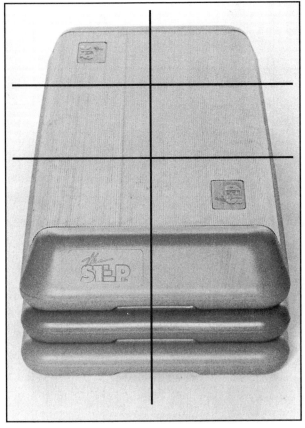

ARM GESTURES TO STEP #:

1. _____
2. _____
3. _____
4. _____
5. _____
6. _____
7. _____
8. _____
9. _____
10. _____
11. _____
12. _____
13. _____
14. _____
15. _____
16. _____
17. _____
18. _____
19. _____
20. _____

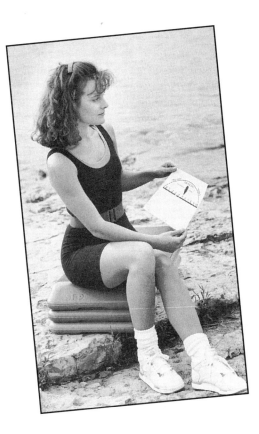

9

Stress Management Principles and Relaxation Techniques

Committing yourself to permanently anchor a mindset for fitness is an exciting goal. Experiencing personal excellence in any or all of the dimensions of your life requires you to become more aware of your potential. To understand potential and unlimited possibilities, we each must begin by setting a *standard* — establishing a starting point or basis — from which to grow. Your stress in balance or a balanced state of well-being expresses this ideal condition. By taking apart this abstract concept and labeling is parts, you will come to understand just how to initiate the process. This will lead to your managing the most productive and rewarding results imaginable in any and all of the dimensions of your life.

ESTABLISHING THE FOUNDATION

All of our world and universe is based on balance. Personal wellness is your life in balance. It requires actions, emotions, attitudes, beliefs, your will, and your power-source, all kept in mind and utilized in solving problems. Life balance or *wellness* is illustrated in Figure 9.1 as six components or balls that we need to keep juggling in the air, all at once. These six components are: physical, emotional, social, spiritual, intellectual, and talent expression. Each of these six components is an equally important contributor to the total balancing act we must engage in every day.

When any wellness component being juggled and kept in balance gets overlooked temporarily,

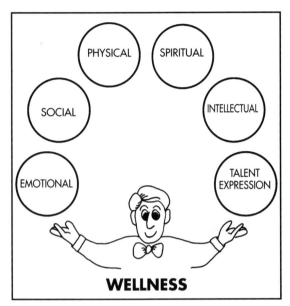

Figure 9.1. Wellness is achieved by balancing six key dimensions of your life.

Developing a working definition for *success* — knowing when you've achieved this balance — is one way. Take some quiet time to develop your own definition for success. Ask yourself "What is balance in my life?"

■   ■   ■

*Success is the ongoing process of
striving and growing to become more,
in each of the dimensions of wellness,
while positively contributing to others' needs.*

■   ■   ■

You can unconditionally believe that you are successful in anything you attempt in life if you (a) attempt and grow from it; (b) make more distinctions about what you're doing, and (c) accomplish it for the purpose of positively contributing what you've learned to others. By adopting this definition for success, it is difficult to feel like a loser or failure.

Consider the points mentioned as steps in a journey rather than as a destination. Life is an ongoing process, and wellness and success are landmarks in the journey. There is no one port or station in life — no one place to arrive at — once and for all. The true joy of life is the trip! A port or station evokes a mental image to be held in expectation so we can tap our unlimited potential in creative problem-solving. Life must be lived and enjoyed in the present moment as accomplished steps, as we go along. The final port will come along soon enough.

or forgotten totally, it falls out of this balanced alignment and drops out of sight. We are then out of sync with life or get the feeling of not being whole. This is understandable, because we aren't. We've allowed one component or several components of our lives to take over and receive all of our attention.

For example, if the expression of our talent (our job or career pursuit, or volunteering) takes an inordinate amount of our mental and physical energy every day, little time is left to participate in a physical fitness program, to develop a social network of friends, and to intellectually pursue other interests that can provide positive release of stress. Our physical, social, or intellectual ball drops and is forgotten. We soon experience the results: a decline in physical fitness, loss of a well-rounded social network of friends, or a boring, one-dimensional focus in our daily conversations.

SUCCESS

How do we know if and when we are truly balancing all of these six areas of our lives?

BALANCING THE SIX WELLNESS DIMENSIONS

Each component or dimension of wellness — each ball we juggle — has specific themes that are explored in this text, either lightly or in-depth. The *physical wellness* component is exemplified by a regular program of the physical expenditure of energy for increasing one's flexibility, heart and lung capacity, and muscular strength and endurance; maintaining a good body position (good posture) while exerting this physical effort; selecting a proper intake, in both variety and amount, of food and liquid; and maintaining a proper body weight (lean-to-fat ratio).

The *emotional wellness* component deals with pleasure and pain (see Figure 9.2). It looks at the distinctions or labels for pleasure (joy) and pain (sadness, anger, fear) and the mixed neuro-associations we feel when these two big emotions are blended (confusion first, then a various assortment and labeling of distinctive others). Becoming aware of the precise emotions we feel, and aware of what we link to pleasure and pain, will assist us in being rational and able to choose productive behavioral responses to life situations.

The *social wellness* component involves creating balance in your time alone and time with others. We can, of course, choose to be independent and achieve every goal we ever set alone.

But you will discover that the most successful and mature people, who regularly tap into their full, unlimited potential, are those persons who are *inter*-dependent. They intentionally choose to interact with other people regularly, even when they could fully accomplish their goals alone. They are able to stretch themselves to unbelievable heights because they constantly draw upon other people as their key resources.

Another theme in the social wellness component involves becoming aware of your communication skills. Sharpening your assertiveness and confrontational skills with others will assist you in becoming a victor instead of a victim in life.

The *intellectual wellness* component challenges you to become a lifelong learner, and to never become complacent and satisfied with past learning and accomplishments. Keeping an open mind to growth and change in the world at large will help us realize that our potential, individually

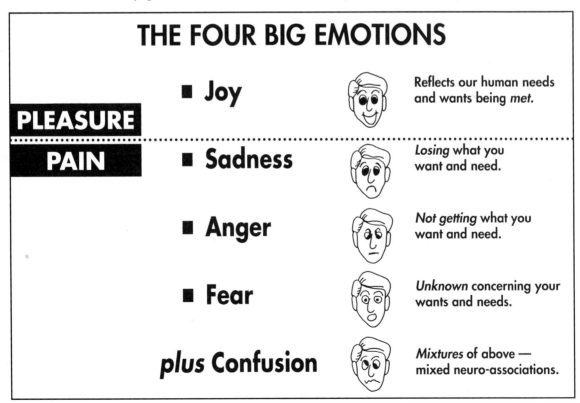

Figure 9.2. The four big emotions.

and collectively, has no boundaries. The only boundaries or limits to our potential are the ones we self-impose inside our heads.

The *spiritual wellness* component challenges you to investigate the balance between relying on your own self-energy source (willpower) and that which ultimately "fuels" you. Finding purpose or the meaning of your existence is assisted by developing a belief system, expressed as philosophies by which you live your life daily.

The *talent expression* component is the sixth dimension of wellness to keep in balance. Your talents are your natural and trained abilities and interests that become translated into your career path or jobs, the volunteer giving of your time to others, and many times the activities you engage in to relieve your stress (stress outlets). Because it usually has a significant impact on self-worth and prestige, this is probably one of the most difficult components for us to keep in perspective and balanced with the other five dimensions of wellness.

Our Four Basic Needs

Why do we want to keep our wellness in balance — for what reasons, purposes, intentions? The four clearly defined survival *needs* we all must have met, supported by the wellness components of our lives, are:

1. I need to live and be healthy.
2. I need to be loved.
3. I need prestige (self-worth) and power (the ability to take action).
4. I need variety and change in my life.

These needs are *birthrights* that we all require for survival and should never be taken away or used as avenues by which to manipulate others.

In addition to our four basic needs[1] is our wide variety of wants. Our *wants* are the privileges or extra comforts we attempt to attain by being responsible and accountable for the actions we take in life. We should begin to label not only what we require for survival (our *needs*, which we also call our ends or ultimate goals) but also what

gives us additional pleasure and joy in the process (our *wants*, also called the means to our ends, or our time priorities). When we clearly understand both our basic needs and our desires or wants, we can pinpoint the purposes of and intentions for our various wellness decisions.

Balance In Brief

The foundation of life is grounded in balance or a *wellness state*, composed of six dimensions: physical, emotional, social, spiritual, intellectual, and talent expression. Developing an all-encompassing definition for success in life provides us with the opportunity to measure and know if and when we achieve individual life balance of the six wellness components. Developing this balance will satisfy our survival needs as well as our additional pleasure-filled wants.

What happens when we become imbalanced and stress enters our life? We must be realistic and aware that life will not be a continual, perfect balance for us, for life is not static and unchanging. Change is a constant. Thus we must consider how to deal with imbalance in our life.

STRESS: DEFINED AND MANAGED

Demands. Problems. Challenges. Change. Whatever you choose to call it, *imbalance* happens within the journey of life. We cannot control our world and all it presents to us. Drunk drivers permanently injure us. Fire and floods destroy our homes and belongings. Death takes our loved ones. A close friend permanently moves far away. We win the lottery. Imbalance asserts itself daily and throughout our life, and we are left to react. *Stress* is our response. We cannot control the changes, demands, problems, or even the dirty deals we encounter, but we can learn how to manage certain situations so they are less offensive to us.

Probably the most noted scientific researcher in modern times on the topic of stress and its effect on the human body is the late Viennese-born endocrinologist, Hans Selye. In his words:

> **Stress is the non-specific response of the body to any kind of demand that is made upon it.[2]**

Physiological Responses To Stress

The physiological response of your body to the positive or negative stressful demands impinging upon it from life situations includes:

- Increased sugar in the blood
- Increased rate of breathing
- Faster heart rate
- Higher blood pressure
- Activation of the blood-clotting mechanism to mitigate effects of injury
- Increased muscle tension
- Cessation of digestion, and diversion of blood to brain and muscles
- More perspiration output
- Decreased salivation
- Loosening of bladder and bowel muscles
- Outpouring of various hormones, including adrenalin
- Dilation of pupils of the eyes
- Heightening of all your senses.

In effect, your body goes into a "Red Alert" and you are ready to fight or flee. This has thus been named the *fight or flight* response to stress.

Many times you can't do either — fight or flee. You must stay in the situation and "stew." If this response, as characterized by the above list, is long enough or severe enough, you experience wear and tear on your bodily systems. This leaves you open to the invasion of some sort of illness.

Once a person becomes ill, the illness also becomes a stressor. This increases your stress response (again, as described in the list of bodily changes) and you are caught in a double-bind.[3]

Good or bad, stress is our response to any kind of imbalancing resulting from demands, problems, challenges, or changes. Therefore, scientifically and physiologically, stress is a *neutral* term. Positive stress, called *eustress*, is exemplified by running a marathon or seeing our loved one after seven months at war. Negative stress, called *distress*, occurs, for example, when we experience a car accident or our home being vandalized. The goal in managing either kind of stress is the same as with all of life: to achieve a balanced state. This can be more easily understood using an analogy.

Stress management can be compared to playing a guitar. To play the guitar, we must use strings that come in a package, limp and with no tension on them (no demands or challenges). If there is no tension or stress on the strings, we can make no sounds. The same comparison goes for our lives. If we have no stress, we have no challenges, no risks, no growth. Life is boring, and so are we, because there is just not enough going on in our life. But stretch those strings to their potential by playing them on the instrument with just the right amount of tension on them, add the human touch, and we will make beautiful sounds — harmony. Place too much tension on the strings (too many commitments on our time), and even the slightest pressure will cause the strings to pop — and so will we.

To experience life with continual growth, imbalance must occur to create room for new possibilities. Change is one of the certainties of life. It is a given. If we approach change from a positive perspective, it can open the doors to unlimited possibilities and growth. If we take the negative view and see it as a threat to our comfortable stability, change can imprison us in the depths of despair and result in stagnation. The choice of perspective, and our subsequent reactions, is ours to make.

Coping Skills

How have you chosen to use your resources in the past to cope (regain balance) when life has dealt you an imbalancing experience? Have you begun to realize that to stay mentally balanced, we all do *something* to cope with the stress in our lives? Some of these coping mechanisms are positive, and some are negative and detrimental to our total well-being. How do you habitually cope with stress? What are your positive means, and what are your negative, detrimental means? Establish a goal to work on now, to improve the one response to stress that seems most disabling to you.

You probably will come away from this reflection a lot less judgmental of other people and their abilities to cope with stress. Knowing that we all do something to relieve and cope with the stress in our lives can help you tolerate another person's choices that sometimes directly affect you. You come away realizing that some people are not *bad* people because, say, they smoke cigarettes, but are simply making a *bad choice* in coping with the stress in their lives.

Your success in adjusting to and managing your response to stress can provide you with growth and increased confidence to meet your next challenge (life situation). We each learn how to adjust to everyday big and small problems and life situations by using our vast internal resources. We are not born adjusted; we systematically learn our adjustments.

Stress/Time/Life Management

You can learn many effective strategies to manage stress. Developing your ability to relax is among the most important. Two guided imagery techniques are suggested to follow the positive stress of your workout hour or to relieve the negative stresses you encounter every day. Each takes only a few minutes to visualize. If you use both techniques at one time, you will experience a *cumulative effect*, a deeper relaxation, perhaps even culminating in sleep.

Choose what result you desire. You may wish to simply enhance a workout with one brief relaxation technique lasting 3 minutes, to successfully

lower your heart rate and breathing, cease sweating profusely, and curb other physiologies. Or you may want to rejuvenate yourself for 10 minutes during a busy day by refocusing your attention before a big event such as an exam, speech, athletic contest, or interview, by using both techniques. At bedtime you may choose to totally relax to the point at which you go directly to sleep, which may entail both of these techniques, plus others you develop.

Two successful methods for using these techniques are:

1. Having someone cue you by reading them slowly;

2. Recording them slowly onto a cassette tape, then playing them to relax.

Enjoy these classic guided-imagery techniques and then develop more imagery of your own. Take a trip to your favorite vacation spot or re-experience talking to the heroes and role models in your life.

■ ■ ■

Ease the pounding of your heart
by the quieting of your mind.

■ ■ ■

GUIDED IMAGERY
1 Total Body Scanning

This technique utilizes your powers of control through your imagination. Your mind seeks out and recognizes tension and eliminates it through your ability to imagine the relaxation. It requires no physical exertion or planned tensing of muscle groups. Total body scanning has four steps: establishing the position; establishing the breathing pattern; tuning in to various parts of the body; and heart rate monitoring followed by simple static stretching to make you alert again (unless the technique is used prior to going to sleep).

Step 1: Relaxation Position

■ Lie on your back. If you feel uncomfortable because your entire back is not in contact with the floor, raise one knee up with your foot flat on the floor approximately 1 foot from your buttocks (see Figure 9.3). Individuals with substantial buttocks or shoulder mass will find that this knee-up position will relieve the arched lower back feeling.

■ Turn your head slightly to one side. When you become totally relaxed, your tongue will relax backward and cover your windpipe if you keep your head straight in line with the rest of you.

■ Place your arms on the floor at your sides, palms down, with elbows slightly bent. Flexed joints are more relaxed.

■ Place your legs apart (not crossed or in contact with one another). As the legs relax your feet will tend to roll outward.

■ If you relax best with your eyes open, keep them open. If you relax best with your eyes closed, close them. If you keep them open, focus continuously on one object only.

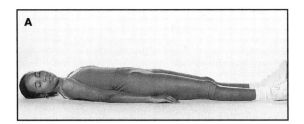

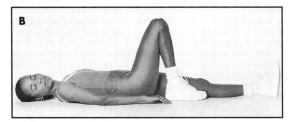

Figure 9.3. Relaxation positions.

Step 2: Deep Breathing

■ Take a deep breath and hold it in your lungs. Focus on the stretched-tight feeling you get in your chest by holding in the oxygen.

■ Now, slowly and purposefully, breathe out (through puckered lips), a long, steady exhale. Create an image in your mind to lengthen the exhale. For example, see yourself blowing the fuzzy seeds off of a dandelion that has gone to seed or blowing a long, steady note on a flute.

■ Repeat this inhale, holding it, and follow with another slow, steady, long exhale. During this inhalation and exhalation, recognize that these next few minutes belong only to you. Do not share them with anybody or anything. Whatever problems, worries, or cares you have, including whatever you are going to do next in your day, briefly think what they are and list them all by writing them on a mental chalkboard in your mind. Then, again mentally, take out a big chalk eraser and wipe each of them off, one at a time, so you are looking at a blank chalkboard in your mind. Verbalize a thought to yourself (e.g., "This is my time now and you [problem] are just going to have to wait"). Then forget it during your relaxation technique!

■ Now follow your breathing cycle, whether it is fast, slow, regular, or irregular. Mentally tune in and follow each inhale and each exhale. Picture yourself on an elevator wherein each exhale is a ride down one more floor (each inhale is the brief pause for the floor stop, door opening and closing. Or imagine that your mind is on a slow roller coaster ride of up and down, up and down.

■ As you begin to relax, the exhalation (breathing out) becomes longer and longer. Don't interfere with your inhalation and exhalation. Ride with it and experience the longer ride out. This begins true relaxation.

■ At various times during the entire body scanning relaxation technique, you will have to mentally tune back in to your breathing technique, for mastering this "elevator ride" is the central focus of your relaxation.

Step 3: Tuning In

■ Start at the top of your head, travel down to the tips of your toes, and return to your midsection.

■ On the top of your head, mentally feel the "part" of your hair. Make it wide by relaxing your scalp.

■ Mentally envision your ears. Drop all tension to your ears. If you are wearing earrings, mentally feel them as heavy on your earlobes.

■ Tune in to your forehead. Is it tense and full of wrinkles? Make it flat and wide with no wrinkles. Picture it smooth and shiny.

■ What is the space between your eyebrows doing? Is it grooved and full of wrinkles? Relax. Make a wide space between your eyebrows. This is one of the telltale locations of human stress. A person who is highly stressed seems to permanently tense the space between the eyebrows (contracted, wrinkled). Calm, serene people stand out because this small space is wide, relaxed, and untensed.

■ Relax your eyebrows as if heavy weights were pulling down the ends. This also will relax your temple area.

■ A hinge joint near your ear hole opens and closes your lower jaw. Relax that mandible joint by dropping your lower jaw. It will make your lips part. Relax your chin.

■ When you relax your jaw, mentally feel your teeth and tongue. When some people try to practice total relaxation, they tightly press (tense) their tongue to the roof of their mouths. Also, many people grit or grind their teeth at night, an audible sign of tension in the area.

■ Relax your throat by thinking of the feeling you get with the second stage of swallowing.

People who sing or play wind instruments have been trained in this technique to relax the area so the best sounds will come out of a relaxed vocal mechanism.

■ Drop your shoulders and chest to make a wide space between your ears and shoulders. We unnecessarily unconsciously tense this area throughout the day. Whether we drive a car or walk in miserable weather, we tense the shoulders up near our ears, encouraging neckaches and headaches. When you think about it next time, untense these muscles if you don't actually need to hold them in a tensed manner.

■ Allow the weight of your chest to sink through to the floor. Think: heavy chest.

■ Drop all tension from your upper arms, elbows, lower arms, and hands until you can just feel your fingertips pulsating on the floor. You may feel a tingling in your fingertips.

■ Relax your buttocks. This is the key to untensing the lower half of your body.

■ Relax your kneecaps. This joint connects your upper and lower leg, and many times we tense the knee area when we attempt to relax other body parts. When you relax the knees, the upper legs will relax and the heavy weight of your legs will begin to drop to the floor. Likewise, the lower legs respond almost automatically, with the feet rolling outward.

■ Mentally feel what your toes are doing. Are they tensed and curled under? If so, stretch them out and then relax them.

■ Now return to the most difficult place to relax — the stomach and intestinal area. Focus your mind on the navel area and picture a wide, flat, picturesque pond. Envision a small pebble being tossed into the very center, creating a soft, rippling effect in which each ripple is a wave of relaxation. Feel the weight of your navel area sinking through, past your spine, onto the floor below you.

■ Return to your breathing cycle, and follow it several times. Focus totally on the long, slow exhale.

■ Now just rest a few moments and enjoy the totally untensed feeling.

Step 4: Heart Rate Monitoring and Stretch

■ In this lying-down position, feel for your pulse. Mentally picture and feel your heart beating. Actively try to slow it down with your mind. Cue it to beat slower.

■ Count your pulse for 15 seconds and multiply by 4 for a minute heart rate count. How does this compare with your resting heart rate count after 6–8 hours of sleep? What does 3 minutes of relaxation do for your body's recovery from exercise or daily stress?

■ Before you get up, sit up slowly and stretch your arms, legs, chest, and back, so you become alert immediately. You must do this 15-second stretch or you'll find yourself yawning for an hour afterward! Of course, if you do this relaxation procedure before going to bed, omit this stretch.

2 The Control Panel with One Large Dial

This second guided imagery technique has been found to be one of the easiest to visualize and integrate into a personal fitness program involving change. (If you will recall, the control panel was used earlier to rate perceived exertion.) The control panel (Figure 9.4), presented at the end of this chapter, is used now for rating, or quantifying, levels of tension and relaxation you feel within your body.

First, give a concrete label to each number on the control panel, from 0–10, as to what that level of relaxation/tension represents to you. Maybe 0 represents totally relaxed inner peace or lying on a warm beach, 5 represents balance and peak performances, and 10 means totally out

of control or experiencing death, disease, or divorce. Write entries for what each number represents to you. Then give today's best/worst moments a number. Now that you have the idea of quantifying stress, visualize this second guided imagery technique.

■ Visualize yourself in a safe place that represents relaxation to you, possibly your bedroom. Envision yourself there, seated in front of a control panel that has one large dial.[3] Continue to hold onto that image in your mind's eye for the duration of the technique, and soon you will feel as if you were actually there.

■ This large dial can be turned to any setting from 0 to 10, which represents all the levels of relaxation and tension you are able to experience. Zero represents all of the relaxation that's possible for you to feel, and 10 represents as much tension as you are able to experience at one time.

■ Begin to look closely at this dial that directly monitors and controls the level of tension in your body. What is the reading on the dial at this moment (from 0 to 10)?

■ See yourself reaching over to turn it down. See yourself turning that dial down, v-e-r-y s-l-o-w-l-y, a little bit at a time. Feel your body relaxing more and more as you turn it down.

■ Feel the tension in your body lessening more and more as you turn the dial all the way down. As all of the tension in your body ebbs away, turn the dial all the way down to zero. Your entire body is just as relaxed as it possibly can be. All of your previous tension is replaced with peaceful feelings of total relaxation and a centered calmness. Currents of gentle tranquillity soothe every muscle, every nerve, every fiber of your being.

■ Return now to the moment in your day and the location where you were prior to your relaxation. Open your eyes and enjoy a fresh, new beginning.

From now on, relax just like this, whenever you choose, by sitting or lying down, closing your eyes for a few moments, and visualizing yourself turning down the dial on this control panel. The more you practice this new ability, the more easily and the more deeply you'll be able to relax, and the longer these feelings of relaxation will remain with you.

You'll be able to sleep better at night, awaken more refreshed, work more efficiently without being bothered by people or situations during the day, feel rejuvenated to perform your very best when you need to, and enjoy your leisure time activities to the fullest. Your unlimited potential awaits you in every aspect of your life. Whether it be rest, work, or leisure, every aspect of your life will be considerably improved and enriched by your new ability to relax whenever you choose.

SUMMARY

Life is a journey of many steps. We desire the pleasure that balance gives to us. We attempt to find ways to manage when imbalance (stress) enters the scene. A most enjoyable means of regaining the balance we seek is through relaxation techniques, of which there are many possibilities. This chapter presents the popular form of relaxation techniques called guided imagery. It focuses on developing an awareness of our own personalized resources which we have stored within, to manage the stress of our lives, through two techniques: total body scanning and the control panel with one large dial.

The blueprint for mastery has been drawn. Practice is what will permanently program the management of your stress.

The Control Panel with One Large Dial

RELAXED

CONTROL DIAL

Use as relaxation ▼ strategy

TENSED

| 0 | 1 | 2 | 3 | 4 | 5 | 6 | 7 | 8 | 9 | 10 |

- PEAK Performances.
- "Balance."

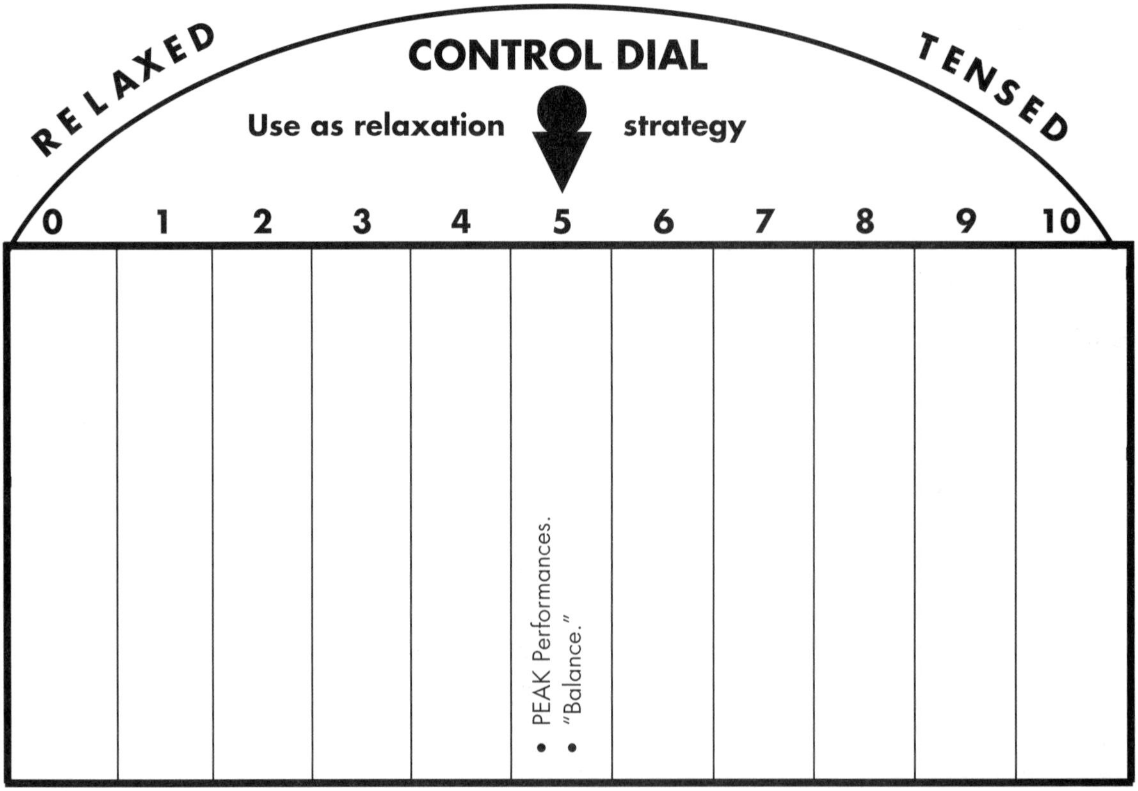

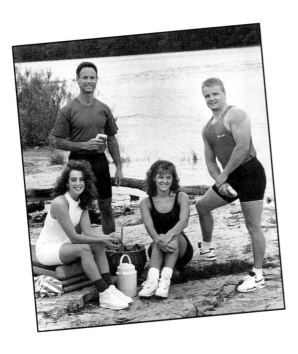

10

Eating For Fitness

"Choose what is best; habit will soon render it agreeable and easy." Ancient philosopher Pythagoras stated this principle of making choices many years ago and it hasn't really changed today. Better or best choices are available for you to make. The actions you take, based on the best information you can get, will become blueprinted and your mindset will be established for making fitness choices.

diet does not properly provide them, your body cannot perform well, mentally or physically.

This is where choice comes in. You may know what the better choices of foods are (called *nutrient dense* foods[1]), but if you don't eat the best choices available to you, you really don't know good nutrition at all. Good health, optimum fitness, and good nutrition result from not just knowing what is best, but choosing it 80 to 90% of the time.[2]

EATING FOR FITNESS

Your body has two basic types of nutrient needs:

- Foods that satisfy your energy needs.
- Foods that meet the needs for growth, repair, and regulation of body processes.

Nutrients are chemical substances that your body absorbs from food during digestion. Your body needs at least 40 nutrients. *Diet* here means total intake of food and drink. Essential nutrients are those your body cannot make or is unable to make in adequate amounts. These nutrients must be obtained from what you eat and drink. If your

BEST CHOICES FOR A BALANCED DIET

A well-balanced diet is one that contains the following six basic nutrients. Proper amounts of each are established according to your age, gender, activity level, and state of wellness:

- Carbohydrates
- Fats
- Proteins
- Vitamins
- Minerals
- Water

These nutrients can be supplied from one of two eating plans presented here: (a) *Food Guide Pyramid, A Guide to Daily Food Choices*, established by the U. S. Department of Agriculture,[3] and shown in Figure 10.1, or (b) the four food groups as illustrated in the pamphlet "Guide to Good Eating," published by the National Dairy Council,[4] and shown in Figures 10.2–10.5. *The eating plan described throughout this chapter follows the guidelines presented in the latter plan.*

You cannot always take in all of the essential nutrients every 24 hours. What *is* important is that over a span of several days and weeks, you continually select from the four groups to meet nutrient needs.

NUTRIENT DENSITY

Following the figures of each food group shown here, foods have been listed according to *nutrient density, the amount of nutrition per calorie each food provides.* To get the most nutrition for the least calories, choose foods from the four-star groups.[5] The categories are:[6]

4 stars = most nutrition per calorie

3 stars = next to most nutrition per calorie

2 stars = next to least nutrition per calorie

1 star = least nutrition per calorie.

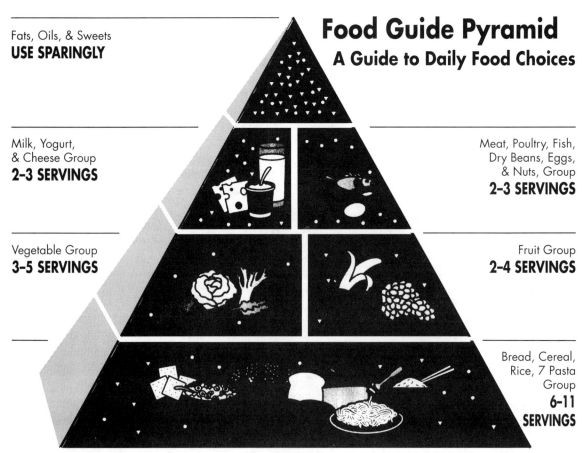

Food Guide Pyramid
A Guide to Daily Food Choices

Fats, Oils, & Sweets
USE SPARINGLY

Milk, Yogurt, & Cheese Group
2-3 SERVINGS

Meat, Poultry, Fish, Dry Beans, Eggs, & Nuts, Group
2-3 SERVINGS

Vegetable Group
3-5 SERVINGS

Fruit Group
2-4 SERVINGS

Bread, Cereal, Rice, 7 Pasta Group
6-11 SERVINGS

Figure 10.1. Food guide pyramid: A guide to daily food choices.[3]

From U. S. Department of Agriculture

If you know little about human physiology (how your vital processes work), it's best not to resort to chance or whatever nutritional guidelines you encounter. An abundance of scientifically-based, easy-to-read, literature has been researched with controls and explains what is entailed in balancing the needed basic nutrients. Select guidelines developed by well-established medical and fitness professionals rather than those from your favorite movie and television stars or supermarket trade magazines.

Milk Group

The only group in which the serving sizes change in reference to your age is the milk group.

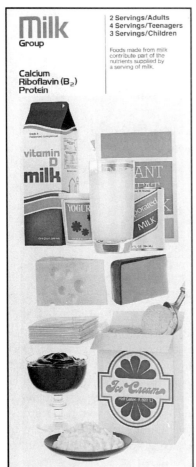

Figure 10.2.
Milk group.

Rating:	Food Choices in Ranked Order:	Serving:
****	nonfat plain yogurt,	
	nonfat milk,	1 cup (8 oz.)
	lowfat cheese,	1 ounce
	buttermilk, lowfat plain	
	yogurt, 1%-2% milk	1 cup (8 oz.)
***	regular fat cheese,	
	ricotta cheese,	1 ounce
	whole milk, kefir, lowfat	
	yogurt w/fruit,	1 cup
	lowfat chocolate milk,	
	nonfat frozen yogurt	1 cup
**	pudding, custard	1 cup
	lowfat frozen yogurt,	
	ice milk	1½ cups
*	cottage cheese	2 cups
	milkshake	1½ cups
	Kissle	1 cup
	ice cream	1½ cups

Note: Nutrient density figured for **calcium.**

Adults need two servings except: pregnant or lactating women need four servings; growing, pre-adolescent children need three servings; and teen-agers need four servings. Calcium, riboflavin (vitamin B_2), and protein are the key nutrients needed to build the basic structure and strength of bones and teeth, assist in the production of energy needs, and help in the growth and maintenance of every living cell. If you are not an avid milk fan, you can eat any of the foods in the milk group and it will supply the calcium, riboflavin, and protein you need.

Meat Group

Even though this group is called the "meat group," plant foods, when eaten together, can supply the needed protein, niacin, iron, and thiamine and are considered an alternative to eating meat.

Some of the plant foods that can be combined so their proteins complement each other (allow the amino acids to combine to form balanced protein) are: dried beans and whole wheat, dried beans and corn or rice, peanuts and wheat.[7]

Everyone needs two servings per day of the meat group (except pregnant women, who need

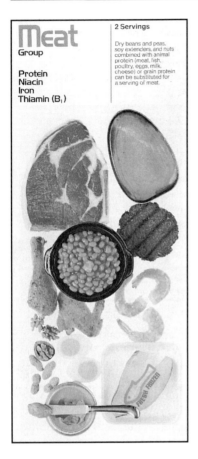

Figure 10.3. Meat group.

three servings per day). One serving is equal to two ounces of cooked lean meat, fish, or poultry, or the protein equivalent. Visually, a 2-ounce portion fills the palm of an average hand and is the width of the little finger.

Cheeses are counted as servings of meat or milk, but not simultaneously. All excess fat should be removed from any meat you eat. You should remove the skin from poultry, and eat only the meat, eliminating unnecessary calories.

Fruit and Vegetable Group

This group provides vitamins A and C, which are actually catalysts or action starters. The most important functions are:

- Forms and maintains skin and body linings.
- Cements substances to promote strength in cells and hasten healing of injuries.
- Functions in all visual processes.
- Aids in the use of iron.

Everyone needs four servings per day. One serving is equivalent to:

- Medium size whole fruit or vegetable
- 1 cup raw
- 1/2 cup cooked
- 1/2-3/4 cup juice
- 1/4 cup dried fruit

Sources of Vitamin A

Orange and green. Remembering two simple colors will help you remember that foods of these colors will provide Vitamin A. Dark green, leafy, or orange vegetables and fruits (such as carrots, sweet potatoes, and greens) should be eaten at least every other day . Because vitamin A is stored in the fat tissue of the body, an overdose through supplementation in pill form can be fatal. (The same is true for the other fat-soluble vitamins — D, E, and K.)

Rating:	Food Choices in Ranked Order:	Serving:
★★★★	lean cuts of: beef, veal, fish, pork, lamb, poultry (visible fat removed)	2-3 ounces, cooked
	eggs	2
★★★	regular and higher fat cuts of: beef, fish, pork, lamb, poultry, (visible fat **not** removed);	2-3 ounces cooked
	tofu	7 ounces
	dried beans, peas, lentils	1 cup cooked
★★	nuts and seeds	½ cup
★	peanut butter	4 tbsp.
	hot dog, luncheon meats, sausage	2-3 ounces

Note: Nutrient density figured for **iron** and **protein**.

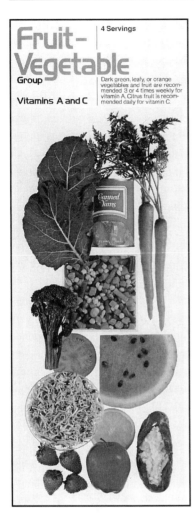

Figure 10.4.
Fruit and
vegetable group.

Rating:	Food Choices in Ranked Order:
****	spinach, chard, broccoli, cantaloupe, tomatoes, brussels sprouts, asparagus, kale, green peppers, winter squash, romaine lettuce
***	vegetable juice, zucchini, green beans, oranges, cabbage, cauliflower, sweet potatoes, apricots, cucumbers, orange juice, carrots, grapefruit, celery
**	artichokes, strawberries, peas, corn, bananas, potatoes, beets, peaches, iceberg lettuce, sprouts, mushrooms, pears, avocados, pineapple juice
*	apples, raisins, grapes, canned fruit, dried fruit, french fries

Note: Nutrient density figured for **folic acid, Vitamins A and C.**

Sources of Vitamin C

Fruits and vegetables such as broccoli, oranges, grapefruits, and strawberries are recommended daily for supplying the needed catalyst, vitamin C. This vitamin is water-soluble, which means that if too much is taken in, the excess is excreted through the urine. If you decide to take vitamin C supplement pills in massive doses, your body reacts by increasing the level it needs. If you then suddenly stop taking vitamin C supplements, your body reacts as if it were deficient! Supplementation is costly and unnecessary for well people who eat properly.

Grain Group (Whole, Fortified, Enriched)

Although this group assists with the growth and maintenance of cells and with the elimination process (fiber provides bulk to your waste for

Rating:	Food Choices in Ranked Order:	Serving:
****	bran (1/3 cup) and whole grain (1 cup) cereals,	1/3-1 cup ready-to-eat or 1/2 cup cooked;
	whole wheat breads and rolls,	1 slice or 1/2 bun;
	whole grain crackers,	4
	corn tortillas	1
***	pasta/noodles, brown rice,	1/2 cup
	enriched breads and rolls,	1 slice or 1/2 bun;
	cornbread	2" square
**	flour tortilla	1
	bagel	1/2
	plain muffin	1
	graham and saltine crackers	4
	pancakes	1
	other cereals	1 cup
	granola type cereal	1/3 cup
	pita bread	1/2 pocket
*	breadsticks (3), English muffin (1/2), enriched rice (1/2 cup cooked), biscuit (1), stuffing (1/2 cup cooked), croissant (1/2).	

Note: Nutrient density figured for **fiber.**

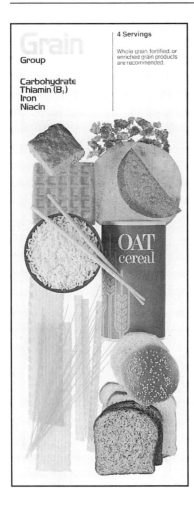

Figure 10.5. Grain group.

fat weight, watch the amount of additional energy food you intake. If, however, you are an active person, such as a varsity or endurance athlete, you will *want* to provide an abundance of this energy food.

Combination Foods

These items comprise more than one food group. They count as servings (or partial servings) from the groups from which they were made. Some of the food choices are: burritos, casseroles, chef salad, hamburgers, lasagna, macaroni and cheese, pizza, soup, stew, tacos. A new product line that presents an exciting choice is the vegetarian "gardenburger,"[8] to be listed under both the grain and protein food groups.

Extras/Others/"Sometimes" Foods

The foods classified as extras have no recommended number of servings. These food choices provide little nutrition and are often high in sugar, salt, fat, and calories. Classified as extras are: alcoholic beverages, bacon, bouillon, butter, cakes, candy, coffee, cookies, condiments, cream, cream cheese, doughnuts, fruit-flavored drinks, gelatin dessert, gravy, honey, jam, jelly, margarine, mayonnaise, non-dairy creamer, olives, onion rings, pickles, pies, popcorn, potato chips, pretzels, salad dressings, sauces, seasonings, sherbet, soft drinks, sour cream, sugar, tea, tortilla chips, vegetable oils.[9]

MONITORING FOOD AND BEVERAGE INTAKE

easy removal), the major function is to provide *energy*. Your number one daily need is energy to perform every daily function from sleeping to aerobics.

Four servings per day is the minimum amount required for all groups. If you do not use this carbohydrate food for the expenditure of energy, for growth and repair, or eliminate it, you wear it as body fat — future energy. It's like constantly carrying around extra gasoline for your car.

A minimum amount of four servings is suggested as a daily intake. A serving is not all you consume or serve yourself at one time but, rather, a measured amount of food. If you wish to lose

Do you eat a wide variety of foods in moderation as shown in the Food Guide Pyramid or as described in detail from the "Super four" food groups? Begin to formulate your eating plan. Start by thinking about what you had to eat today, and record the foods you ate in relation to the appropriate food group.

For a combination food, think about what foods went into it, and list those foods under the appropriate food group. For example, the cheese on a pizza would be recorded in the milk group, the tomatoes and any other vegetables should be recorded in the fruit-vegetable group, and the crust is recorded in the grain group. The ingredients in a combination food may not always count as a full serving from the food group. Think in terms of quantity of servings, along with its nutrient category.

Continue monitoring your intake for one week. How does it measure up to the standards established for a balanced diet with special attention to selecting nutrient-dense foods? If your diet lacks variety, moderation, or foods from one of the food groups, you may not be getting all the nutrients and energy you need.

It's easy to improve your diet if you take it one step at a time. Start by choosing one challenge to work on, come up with a solution, and spend one week trying to correct it. After it's mastered, choose a second eating challenge that needs attention, and continue until you have a well-managed diet.

NUTRITION AND THE ATHLETE

The proper food intake for athletes is the starting point for training or conditioning. The food groups already presented form the *foundation* of the diet recommended for young athletes. This plan serves as the nucleus for meals both in and out of athletic seasons. There is a vast leeway in the choice of foods within each of the food groups. Major deviations from these food groups should be necessary only rarely. Basic nutritional needs of athletes and nonathletes do not differ except in terms of calories.[10]

Total caloric needs vary with individual metabolism and physical activity. An intake of 2,000 calories each day should be the bare minimum allowed for an athlete involved in a vigorous training program. The amount of calories a young male athlete expends in serious training may range as high as 4,000-6,000 calories per day. Calorie intake that exceeds expenditure for basal body functions, for physical activity, and for growth of lean body mass, however, will still form body fat, so pay attention to your training diet.

A pre-game meal should:

■ Support blood sugar levels to avoid hunger sensations.

■ Leave the stomach and upper bowel empty at the time of competition.

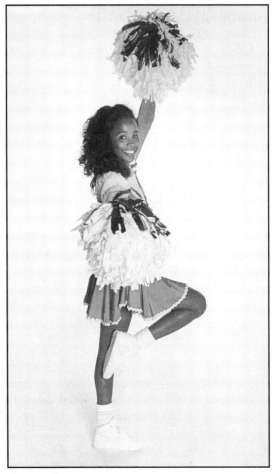

Figure 10.6.

■ Provide maximum hydration.

■ Minimize stomach upset; promote maximum performance.

■ Provide a psychological edge by including foods the athlete likes and believes will make him or her win.

1 *Carbohydrates* in the diet will support blood sugar and provide glycogen stores to maintain these levels. Glycogen, the storage form of carbohydrate, seems to be the quickest and most efficient source of energy.

Good choices of high carbohydrate foods are: apples, applesauce, bagels, baked potatoes, baking powder biscuits, bananas, boiled potatoes, bread, (white, whole wheat), cheese pizza, egg noodles, graham crackers, hard rolls, macaroni and cheese, mashed potatoes, oatmeal, oranges, orange juice, orange sherbet, pancakes (enriched), pears, spaghetti (cooked), sponge cake, sweet potatoes, and waffles.

2 Carbohydrates are digested more rapidly than protein and fat. (A breakfast of toast and jam, cereal with low-fat milk, and fruit or juice will leave the stomach much sooner than a meal of eggs with steak, sausage, or bacon.)

3 Optimum hydration is important to athletes, especially those involved in endurance events, such as long-distance swimming or running. The immediate pre-game diet should consist of 2 to 3 glasses of some beverage, with no less than 8 full glasses each 24 hours.

Whole milk is not recommended because of its high fat content. Caffeine also should be avoided because it may increase nervous tension and agitation before the contest. Non-carbonated fruit drinks are generally a good choice.

4 Concentrated sources of simple sugar such as glucose tablets or undiluted honey should be avoided as they can cause gas distention and

discomfort. Also, bulky foods high in fiber or cellulose are not good choices before an event.

Heavily salted foods probably should be avoided on the day of competition because they can cause water retention, which decreases athletic performance.

5 The pre-game meal should be eaten three to four hours before the contest. For a very demanding sport, a 1,000-calorie meal is ideal. A 500-calorie meal suffices for a sport demanding lower energy.

Athletes make special demands on their bodies and must be physically prepared to meet those demands. The starting block is sound nutrition knowledge and practice. If you sacrifice a winning excellence to an inefficient or harmful diet, reduced strength and endurance and a poor performance will result.

DIETARY GUIDELINES FOR AMERICANS

Food alone cannot make a person healthy, but good eating habits based on moderation and variety can help keep a person healthy and even improve health. The following guidelines suggested for most Americans, developed by the U. S. Department of Agriculture, Health and Human Services, are printed in more detail in the pamphlet, *Nutrition and Your Health: Dietary Guidelines for Americans.*[11] In brief, most Americans need to pay more attention to the following guidelines.

1 *Eat a variety of foods.* No single food supplies all the essential nutrients in the amounts you need. The greater the variety, the less likely you are to develop either a deficiency or an excess of any single nutrient.

2 *Maintain healthy weight.* If you are too fat or too thin, your chances of developing health problems increase (i.e., high blood pressure, diabetes, heart disease, certain cancers). There is no one plan for maintaining healthy weight. If your concern is to lose fat weight, increase your physical activity, eat less fat and fatty foods, eat less sugar and sweets, and avoid too much alcohol.

3 *Choose a diet low in fat, saturated fat, and cholesterol.* If you have a high blood cholesterol level, you have a greater chance of incurring a heart attack. A population such as that of the United States, with diets high in saturated fats and cholesterol, tend to have high blood cholesterol levels.

There is controversy about what recommendations are appropriate for healthy Americans. For the U. S. population as a whole, however, reducing our current intake of total fat, saturated fat, and cholesterol is sensible.

- Choose lean meats, fish, poultry, dry beans, and peas as your protein sources.

- Moderate your intake of eggs and organ meats (such as liver).

- Limit your intake of butter, cream hydrogenated margarines, shortenings, coconut oil, and foods made from those products.

- Trim excess fat off meats.

- Broil, bake, and boil rather than fry.

- Read labels carefully to determine amounts and types of fat and cholesterol in foods.

- Consume 300 mg/day or less of cholesterol.

- Limit fat to 30% of daily calories or less. To determine the percentage of calories in a product that come from fat: 1 gram of fat equals 9 calories. Multiply the grams of fat in a serving times 9. The result equals the number of calories from fat in a serving. Divide the fat calories by the total calories in a serving to determine the percent.

For example, if a chili label reads 1 cup serving = 200 calories/Fat 10 gm/Carbohydrate 5 gm/Sodium 980 mg.: There are 10 grams of fat in 1 cup of chili. 10 grams of fat $\times$ 9 calories = 90 calories from fat in 1 cup. 90 $\div$ 200 = 45% of the calories in 1 cup of chili come from fat![12]

4 *Include plenty of vegetables, fruits, and grain products in your diet.* The major sources of energy in the average U. S. diet are carbohydrates and fats. Carbohydrates have an advantage over fats: They contain less than half the number of calories per ounce than fats.

Complex carbohydrate foods are better than simple carbohydrates. Simple carbohydrates (sugars) provide calories for energy but little else in the way of nutrients. Complex carbohydrates (beans, nuts, fruits, whole-grain breads) contain many essential nutrients plus calories for energy.

Increasing your consumption of certain complex carbohydrates also can increase dietary fiber, which tends to reduce the symptoms of chronic constipation, diverticulosis, and some types of irritable bowel. There is also concern that diets low in fiber content might also increase the risk of developing cancer of the colon. Eating fruits, vegetables, and whole-grain breads and cereals will provide adequate fiber in the diet.

5 *Use sugars only in moderation.* The major hazard from eating too much sugar is tooth decay. The risk increases the more frequently you eat sugar and sweets, especially between meals, if you eat foods that stick to the teeth (sticky candy, dates) and if you consume soft drinks throughout the day.

- Use less of all sugars (white, brown, raw, honey, and syrups).

- Select fresh fruit or fruit canned without heavy syrup.

- Read food labels for sugar included: sucrose, glucose, maltose, dextrose, lactose, fructose, syrup. If it's listed as one of the first ingredients, it has a lot of sugar.

To determine how many teaspoons of sugar a product contains, 5 grams of sugar equal 1 teaspoon. Divide the grams in a serving by 5. For example, if a cereal box label reads 1-cup serving = 140 calories/carbohydrates/starch 10 gm/ sucrose 15 gm/fiber 1 gm: There are 15 grams of sucrose in 1 cup of cereal. 15 grams of sucrose ÷ 5 = 3 teaspoons of simple sugar in 1 cup of cereal. Products are healthier when sucrose (simple sugar) amounts are low.[13]

6 *Consume salt and sodium in moderation.* The major hazard posed by excessive sodium is its effect on blood pressure. In populations where high-sodium intake is common, high blood pressure is also common. In populations with low-sodium intake, high blood pressure is rare. Establish preventive measures, such as:

■ Eliminate all salt use at the table.

■ Cook with little or no salt.

■ Select foods that are low in sodium content.

The dietary goal for sodium intake is approximately 2,000–3,000 mg/day. The items in Table 10.1 contain a relatively high sodium content:

TABLE 10.1.
Relatively High Sodium-Content Foods

Food	Serving Size	Mg/Sodium Content
antacid (in water)	1 dose	564 mg.
canned corn	1 cup	384
cottage cheese	4 ounces	457
dill pickle	1	928
ham	3 ounces	1,114
salt	1 tsp.	1,938
tomato sauce	1 cup	1,498

7 *If you drink alcohol, do so in moderation.* Alcoholic beverages tend to be high in calories and low in other nutrients. Heavy drinkers may lose their appetite for foods that contain essential nutrients. Vitamin and mineral deficiencies occur commonly in heavy drinkers because of poor nutrient intake and because alcohol alters absorption and use of some essential nutrients.

One or two drinks daily seem to cause no harm in adults, but even moderate drinkers need to remember that alcohol is a high-calorie, low-nutrient food. If you wish to achieve or maintain ideal weight, alcohol intake must be well monitored. Women should consume no more than one drink a day, and men, no more than two drinks a day. Count as a drink:

■ 12 ounces of regular beer

■ 5 ounces of wine

■ 1½ ounces of distilled spirits (80 proof)[14].

SUMMARY

Diet is an essential facet of total fitness and wellness. Responsible eating plans are available from the sources named in this chapter. The axiom "the *application* of knowledge is power" applies here. Translating established guidelines and principles into practice will prove to be a powerful source of sustenance and energy that will enhance your physical fitness program.

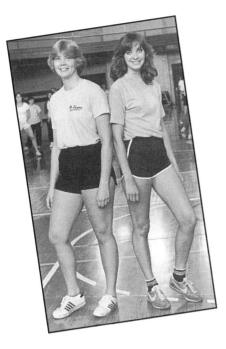

11

Positive Weight Management

Your body is composed of two types of weight: lean weight and fat weight. They are also called lean body mass (or fat-free mass), and fat mass. Lean weight is composed primarily of bones, muscles, and internal organs. It begins to weigh less after maturity when you stop growing at a certain steady pace every year. Fat weight is stored energy and protection for present and future use. The amount of each type of weight you carry is important to know so you can understand what is best for the health of your heart and lungs (cardiorespiratory system).

BODY FAT/BODY LEAN

Body fat can be classified as either essential fat or storage fat. Essential fat is needed for normal physiological functions. Without it, your health begins to deteriorate. This essential fat constitutes about 3% of the total fat in men and 10–12% in women. The percentage is higher in women because it includes gender-related fat such as that found in the breast tissue, the uterus, and other gender-related areas.

Storage fat is the fat stored in adipose tissue, mostly beneath the skin (subcutaneous fat) and around major organs in the body. This fat serves three basic functions:

1. As an insulator to retain body heat;

2. As energy substrate for metabolism;

3. As padding against physical trauma to the body.

The amount of storage fat does not differ between men and women except that men tend to store fat around the waist and women more so around the hips and thighs.[1]

For each individual's amount of lean tissue, a certain percentage of fat can be "worn" to maintain ideal cardiorespiratory efficiency and minimize risk factors associated with heart disease.

You may find that you are perhaps wearing less than a suggested ideal percentage of fat than is listed. This doesn't matter unless you are malnourishing yourself or you cosmetically wish to look heavier. A number of people don't wear ideal percentages. For example, endurance athletes such as marathon runners and Olympic gymnasts both carry much less fat. They burn it off and don't carry the excess. They usually eat right to provide the necessary nutrients and energy and thus display a firm, trim, toned look yet they stay well.

In contrast are individuals who have the starvation disease, anorexia nervosa. They, too, carry less than the suggested ideal percentage of body fat but they do this by also eliminating their lean weight. They desire a trim look but go about it in a way that is against all physiological principles of proper weight loss. To them, weight loss means dropping pounds to be slim at all cost, no matter what kind of weight it is, fat or lean. This is an extremely detrimental way to lose weight. The concept of healthy slimness and unhealthy slimness is elaborated later in the chapter.

DETERMINING YOUR BODY COMPOSITION

"Ideal weight" cannot be determined just by looking at someone. The two college women in the chapter opening photo are both approximately 5′10″ tall and are carrying the same percentage of body fat (28%) on their individual leans. At left, Paula's ideal weight is 145. On the right, Jill's ideal weight is 114.

An assessment of body composition involves determining as precisely as possible an individual's body fat and lean body weight. This enables an accurate estimate of an individual's ideal weight. The traditional standardized weight tables, adjusted for gender, height and frame size, have been shown to be grossly inaccurate for many people. The ideal weight within any one category of these tables can vary up to 22 pounds. Individuals often fall within the normal range for their category but actually can have 10 to 30 pounds of excess body fat.

Measurement techniques now can more accurately determine whether an individual is overweight (overfat) or obese and quantify exactly by how much.

These techniques include:

■ Measuring skinfold thickness

■ Analysis by electrical impedence

■ Underwater weighing (specific gravity)

■ Combine skinfold thickness and anthropometric measures of bone thickness or girth measurements, or both

■ Near-infrared interactance.

Because of the ease of use in an aerobics class setting and the availability of equipment, the first technique is used most often with this population. The fitness component called body composition is assessed, to determine lean weight mass and percentage of body fat. With that information, an estimated ideal body weight can be established that is best for your cardiorespiratory health.

Measuring Skinfold Thickness

Assessment of body composition using skinfold thickness is based on the principle that approximately 50% of the body's fatty tissue is deposited directly beneath the skin. If this tissue is estimated validly and reliably, it can produce a good indication of percent body fat.

This test is done with the aid of a precision instrument called a *skinfold caliper*. Three specific sites must be measured with the calipers and then added together to reflect the total percentage of fat. These measurements may vary slightly on the same subject when they are taken by different professionals. Therefore, pre- and post-measurements preferably should be taken by the same technician.

Using the three-site skinfold testing, the procedure for assessing percent body fat follows:

1. Specific anatomical sites are tested. For men, this is the chest, abdomen, and thigh (Figure 11.1). For women, the triceps, suprailium, and thigh areas are tested (Figure 11.2). All measurements should be taken on the right side of the body with the subject standing. The correct anatomical landmarks for skinfolds are:

Men

Chest: A diagonal fold halfway between the shoulder crease and the nipple.

Abdomen: A vertical fold taken about 1 inch to the right of the umbilicus.

Thigh: A vertical fold on the front of the thigh, midway between the knee and hip.

Women

Triceps: A vertical fold on the back of the upper arm, halfway between the shoulder and the elbow.

Suprailium: A diagonal fold above the crest of the ilium (on the side of the hip).

Thigh: A vertical fold on the front of the thigh, midway between the knee and hip.

2. The technician conducts the measurements by grasping a thickness of skin in the key locations just mentioned, with a thumb and forefinger, and pulling the fold slightly away from the muscular tissue. The calipers are held perpendicular to the fold, and the measurement is taken 1/2 inch below the finger hold. Each site is measured three times, and the values are read to the nearest .1 to .5 mm. The average of the two closest readings is recorded as your final value. The readings are taken in close succession to avoid excessive compression of the skinfold. Releasing and regrabbing the skinfold is required between readings.

3. When doing pre- and post-assessments, the measurement should be conducted at the same time of day. The best time is early in the morning to avoid hydration changes resulting from activity or exercise.

4. The percent fat is obtained by adding all three skinfold measurements and looking up the respective values on Table 11.1 for women, 11.2 for men under forty, and 11.3 for men over forty.

Determining Your Classification

After finding out your percent body fat, you can determine your current body composition classification according to Table 11.4. In this table you will find the health fitness and the high

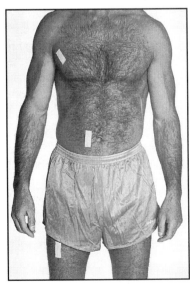

Figure 11.1 Proper anatomical sites for skinfold testing of men.

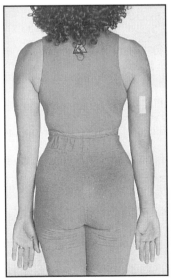

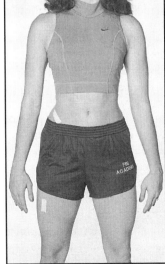

Figure 11.2. Proper anatomical sites for skinfold testing of women.

TABLE 11.1
Percent Fat Estimates for Women Calculated from Triceps, Suprailium, and Thigh Skinfold Thickness

Sum of 3 Skinfolds	Under 22	23 to 27	28 to 32	33 to 37	38 to 42	43 to 47	48 to 52	53 to 57	Over 58
					Age to the Last Year				
23-25	9.7	9.9	10.2	10.4	10.7	10.9	11.2	11.4	11.7
26-28	11.0	11.2	11.5	11.7	12.0	12.3	12.5	12.7	13.0
29-31	12.3	12.5	12.8	13.0	13.3	13.5	13.8	14.0	14.3
32-34	13.6	13.8	14.0	14.3	14.5	14.8	15.0	15.3	15.5
35-37	14.8	15.0	15.3	15.5	15.8	16.0	16.3	16.5	16.8
38-40	16.0	16.3	16.5	16.7	17.0	17.2	17.5	17.7	18.0
41-43	17.2	17.4	17.7	17.9	18.2	18.4	18.7	18.9	19.2
44-46	18.3	18.6	18.8	19.1	19.3	19.6	19.8	20.1	20.3
47-49	19.5	19.7	20.0	20.2	20.5	20.7	21.0	21.2	21.5
50-52	20.6	20.8	21.1	21.3	21.6	21.8	22.1	22.3	22.6
53-55	21.7	21.9	22.1	22.4	22.6	22.9	23.1	23.4	23.6
56-58	22.7	23.0	23.2	23.4	23.7	23.9	24.2	24.4	24.7
59-61	23.7	24.0	24.2	24.5	24.7	25.0	25.2	25.5	25.7
62-64	24.7	25.0	25.2	25.5	25.7	26.0	26.2	26.4	26.7
65-67	25.7	25.9	26.2	26.4	26.7	26.9	27.2	27.4	27.7
68-70	26.6	26.9	27.1	27.4	27.6	27.9	28.1	28.4	28.6
71-73	27.5	27.8	28.0	28.3	28.5	28.8	29.0	29.3	29.5
74-76	28.4	28.7	28.9	29.2	29.4	29.7	29.9	30.2	30.4
77-79	29.3	29.5	29.8	30.0	30.3	30.5	30.8	31.0	31.3
80-82	30.1	30.4	30.6	30.9	31.1	31.4	31.6	31.9	32.1
83-85	30.9	31.2	31.4	31.7	31.9	32.2	32.4	32.7	32.9
86-88	31.7	32.0	32.2	32.5	32.7	32.9	33.2	33.4	33.7
89-91	32.5	32.7	33.0	33.2	33.5	33.7	33.9	34.2	34.4
92-94	33.2	33.4	33.7	33.9	34.2	34.4	34.7	34.9	35.2
95-97	33.9	34.1	34.4	34.6	34.9	35.1	35.4	35.6	35.9
98-100	34.6	34.8	35.1	35.3	35.5	35.8	36.0	36.3	36.5
101-103	35.2	35.4	35.7	35.9	36.2	36.4	36.7	36.9	37.2
104-106	35.8	36.1	36.3	36.6	36.8	37.1	37.3	37.5	37.8
107-109	36.4	36.7	36.9	37.1	37.4	37.6	37.9	38.1	38.4
110-112	37.0	37.2	37.5	37.7	38.0	38.2	38.5	38.7	38.9
113-115	37.5	37.8	38.0	38.2	38.5	38.7	39.0	39.2	39.5
116-118	38.0	38.3	38.5	38.8	39.0	39.3	39.5	39.7	40.0
119-121	38.5	38.7	39.0	39.2	39.5	39.7	40.0	40.2	40.5
122-124	39.0	39.2	39.4	39.7	39.9	40.2	40.4	40.7	40.9
125-127	39.4	39.6	39.9	40.1	40.4	40.6	40.9	41.1	41.4
128-130	39.8	40.0	40.3	40.5	40.8	41.0	41.3	41.5	41.8

Body density is calculated based on the generalized equation for predicting body density of women developed by A. S. Jackson, M. L. Pollock, and A. Ward. *Medicine and Science in Sports and Exercise* 12:175-182, 1980. Percent body fat is determined from the calculated body density using the Siri formula.[1]

TABLE 11.2
Percent Fat Estimates for Men Under 40 Calculated from Chest, Abdomen, and Thigh Skinfold Thickness

				Age to the Last Year				
Sum of 3 Skinfolds	Under 19	20 to 22	23 to 25	26 to 28	29 to 31	32 to 34	35 to 37	38 to 40
8-10	.9	1.3	1.6	2.0	2.3	2.7	3.0	3.3
11-13	1.9	2.3	2.6	3.0	3.3	3.7	4.0	4.3
14-16	2.9	3.3	3.6	3.9	4.3	4.6	5.0	5.3
17-19	3.9	4.2	4.6	4.9	5.3	5.6	6.0	6.3
20-22	4.8	5.2	5.5	5.9	6.2	6.6	6.9	7.3
23-25	5.8	6.2	6.5	6.8	7.2	7.5	7.9	8.2
26-28	6.8	7.1	7.5	7.8	8.1	8.5	8.8	9.2
29-31	7.7	8.0	8.4	8.7	9.1	9.4	9.8	10.1
32-34	8.6	9.0	9.3	9.7	10.0	10.4	10.7	11.1
35-37	9.5	9.9	10.2	10.6	10.9	11.3	11.6	12.0
38-40	10.5	10.8	11.2	11.5	11.8	12.2	12.5	12.9
41-43	11.4	11.7	12.1	12.4	12.7	13.1	13.4	13.8
44-46	12.2	12.6	12.9	13.3	13.6	14.0	14.3	14.7
47-49	13.1	13.5	13.8	14.2	14.5	14.9	15.2	15.5
50-52	14.0	14.3	14.7	15.0	15.4	15.7	16.1	16.4
53-55	14.8	15.2	15.5	15.9	16.2	16.6	16.9	17.3
56-58	15.7	16.0	16.4	16.7	17.1	17.4	17.8	18.1
59-61	16.5	16.9	17.2	17.6	17.9	18.3	18.6	19.0
62-64	17.4	17.7	18.1	18.4	18.8	19.1	19.4	19.8
65-67	18.2	18.5	18.9	19.2	19.6	19.9	20.3	20.6
68-70	19.0	19.3	19.7	20.0	20.4	20.7	21.1	21.4
71-73	19.8	20.1	20.5	20.8	21.2	21.5	21.9	22.2
74-76	20.6	20.9	21.3	21.6	22.0	22.2	23.4	23.0
77-79	21.4	21.7	22.1	22.4	22.8	23.1	23.4	23.8
80-82	22.1	22.5	22.8	23.2	23.5	23.9	24.2	24.6
83-85	22.9	23.2	23.6	23.9	24.3	24.6	25.0	25.3
86-88	23.6	24.0	24.3	24.7	25.0	25.4	25.7	26.1
89-91	24.4	24.7	25.1	25.4	25.8	26.1	26.5	26.8
92-94	25.1	25.5	25.8	26.2	26.5	26.9	27.2	27.5
95-97	25.8	26.2	26.5	26.9	27.2	27.6	27.9	28.3
98-100	26.6	26.9	27.3	27.6	27.9	28.3	28.6	29.0
101-103	27.3	27.6	28.0	28.3	28.6	29.0	29.3	29.7
104-106	27.9	28.3	28.6	29.0	29.3	29.7	30.0	30.4
107-109	28.6	29.0	29.3	29.7	30.0	30.4	30.7	31.1
110-112	29.3	29.6	30.0	30.3	30.7	31.0	31.4	31.7
113-115	30.0	30.3	30.7	31.0	31.3	31.7	32.0	32.4
116-118	30.6	31.0	31.3	31.6	32.0	32.3	32.7	33.0
119-121	31.3	31.6	32.0	32.3	32.6	33.0	33.3	33.7
122-124	31.9	32.2	32.6	32.9	33.3	33.6	34.0	34.3
125-127	32.5	32.9	33.2	33.5	33.9	34.2	34.6	34.9
128-130	33.1	33.5	33.8	34.2	34.5	34.9	35.2	35.5

Body density is calculated based on the generalized equation for predicting body density of men developed by A. S. Jackson, M. L. Pollock. *British Journal of Nutrition* 40:497-504, 1978. Percent body fat is determined from the calculated body density using the Siri formula.[1]

TABLE 11.3
Percent Fat Estimates for Men Over 40 Calculated from Chest, Abdomen, and Thigh Skinfold Thickness

Sum of 3 Skinfolds	Age to the Last Year							
	41 to 43	44 to 46	47 to 49	50 to 52	53 to 55	56 to 58	59 to 61	Over 62
8-10	3.7	4.0	4.4	4.7	5.1	5.4	5.8	6.1
11-13	4.7	5.0	5.4	5.7	6.1	6.4	6.8	7.1
14-16	5.7	6.0	6.4	6.7	7.1	7.4	7.8	8.1
17-19	6.7	7.0	7.4	7.7	8.1	8.4	8.7	9.1
20-22	7.6	8.0	8.3	8.7	9.0	9.4	9.7	10.1
23-25	8.6	8.9	9.3	9.6	10.0	10.3	10.7	11.0
26-28	9.5	9.9	10.2	10.6	10.9	11.3	11.6	12.0
29-31	10.5	10.8	11.2	11.5	11.9	12.2	12.6	12.9
32-34	11.4	11.8	12.1	12.4	12.8	13.1	13.5	13.8
35-37	12.3	12.7	13.0	13.4	13.7	14.1	14.4	14.8
38-40	13.2	13.6	13.9	14.3	14.6	15.0	15.3	15.7
41-43	14.1	14.5	14.8	15.2	15.5	15.9	16.2	16.6
44-46	15.0	15.4	15.7	16.1	16.4	16.8	17.1	17.5
47-49	15.9	16.2	16.6	16.9	17.3	17.6	18.0	18.3
50-52	16.8	17.1	17.5	17.8	18.2	18.5	18.8	19.2
53-55	17.6	18.0	18.3	18.7	19.0	19.4	19.7	20.1
56-58	18.5	18.8	19.2	19.5	19.9	20.2	20.6	20.9
59-61	19.3	19.7	20.0	20.4	20.7	21.0	21.4	21.7
62-64	20.1	20.5	20.8	21.2	21.5	21.9	22.2	22.6
65-67	21.0	21.3	21.7	22.0	22.4	22.7	23.0	23.4
68-70	21.8	22.1	22.5	22.8	23.2	23.5	23.9	24.2
71-73	22.6	22.9	23.3	23.6	24.0	24.3	24.7	25.0
74-76	23.4	23.7	24.1	24.4	24.8	25.1	25.4	25.8
77-79	24.1	24.5	24.8	25.2	25.5	25.9	26.2	26.6
80-82	24.9	25.3	25.6	26.0	26.3	26.6	27.0	27.3
83-85	25.7	26.0	26.4	26.7	27.1	27.4	27.8	28.1
86-88	26.4	26.8	27.1	27.5	27.8	28.2	28.5	28.9
89-91	27.2	27.5	27.9	28.2	28.6	28.9	29.2	29.6
92-94	27.9	28.2	28.6	28.9	29.3	29.6	30.0	30.3
95-97	28.6	29.0	29.3	29.7	30.0	30.4	30.7	31.1
98-100	29.3	29.7	30.0	30.4	30.7	31.1	31.4	31.8
101-103	30.0	30.4	30.7	31.1	31.4	31.8	32.1	32.5
104-106	30.7	31.1	31.4	31.8	32.1	32.5	32.8	33.2
107-109	31.4	31.8	32.1	32.4	32.8	33.1	33.5	33.8
110-112	32.1	32.4	32.8	33.1	33.5	33.8	34.2	34.5
113-115	32.7	33.1	33.4	33.8	34.1	34.5	34.8	35.2
116-118	33.4	33.7	34.1	34.4	34.8	35.1	35.5	35.8
119-121	34.0	34.4	34.7	35.1	35.4	35.8	36.1	36.5
122-124	34.7	35.0	35.4	35.7	36.1	36.4	36.7	37.1
125-127	35.3	35.6	36.0	36.3	36.7	37.0	37.4	37.7
128-130	35.9	36.2	36.6	36.9	37.3	37.6	38.0	38.5

Body density is calculated based on the generalized equation for predicting body density of men developed by A. S. Jackson, M. L. Pollock. *British Journal of Nutrition* 40:497-504, 1978. Percent body fat is determined from the calculated body density using the Siri formula.[1]

TABLE 11.4
Body Composition Classification According to Percent Body Fat

MEN

Age	Excellent	Good	Moderate	Overweight	Obese
<19	12	12.5-17.0	17.5-22.0	22.5-27.0	27.5+
20-29	13	13.5-18.0	18.5-23.0	23.5-28.0	28.5+
30-39	14	14.5-19.0	19.5-24.0	24.5-29.0	29.5+
40-49	15	15.5-20.0	20.5-25.0	25.5-30.0	30.5+
50+	16	16.5-21.5	21.5-26.0	26.5-31.0	31.5+

WOMEN

Age	Excellent	Good	Moderate	Overweight	Obese
<19	17	17.5-22.0	22.5-27.0	27.5-32.0	32.5+
20-29	18	18.5-23.0	23.5-28.0	28.5-33.0	33.5+
30-39	19	19.5-24.0	24.5-29.0	29.5-34.0	34.5+
40-49	20	20.5-25.0	25.5-30.0	30.5-35.0	35.5+
50+	21	21.5-26.5	26.5-31.0	31.5-36.0	36.5+

■ High physical fitness standard

▨ Health fitness standard

From Werner W. K. Hoeger, *Principles & Labs for Physical Fitness & Wellness* (Englewood, CO: Morton Publishing Company, 1991), p. 90.

physical fitness percent fat standards. For example, the recommended health fitness fat percentage for a 20-year-old female is 28% or less. The health fitness standard is established at the point where there seems to be no detriment to health in terms of percent body fat. A high physical fitness range for this same woman would be between 18% and 23%.

The high physical fitness standard does not mean that you cannot be somewhat below this number. As mentioned earlier, many highly trained athletes measurements are below the percentages set. The 3% essential fat for men and 12% for women are the lower limits for people to maintain good health. Below these percentages, normal physiologic functions can be seriously impaired.

In addition, some experts point out that a little storage fat (over the essential fat) is better than none at all. As a result, the health and high fitness standards for percent fat in Table 11.4 are set higher than the minimum essential fat requirements, at a point that is conducive to optimal health and well-being. Also, because lean tissue decreases with age, one extra percentage point is allowed for every additional decade of life.

Your recommended body weight is computed based on the selected health or high fitness fat percentage for your respective age and gender. Your selection of a desired fat percentage should be based on your current percent body fat and your personal health-fitness goals and objectives.

ACHIEVING A HEALTHY SLIMNESS

We seem to readily admit that a primary goal in taking fitness courses is to *appear* healthy and slim. We desire this goal because we can directly see when our body looks nice, lean, and toned; likewise, we can directly see when it looks out of shape and flabby. Many individuals therefore initially focus on a form of "fitness" or "being in shape" that they can readily see.

Your outer appearance , however, is not the entire, or even major, focus of a quality fitness program. You can live without well-toned muscles or a trim figure, but you can't live very long without a strong heart and lungs. Looking attractive and feeling good about your appearance are good ancillary goals. The key word, however, is *healthy* slimness. This will require developing a weight management program that you enjoy following.

PRINCIPLES OF WEIGHT MANAGEMENT

Weight management means controlling the amount of body fat in relation to the amount of lean. Principles of weight management include: *weight maintenance* (keeping the same ratio of fat to amount of lean you're currently carrying); *weight gain* (almost always in terms of lean weight gain, not fat weight gain), and *weight loss* (always in terms of loss of body fat).

Weight Maintenance

In regard to weight maintenance:

■ Your current composition of fat to lean is ideal for your best cardiorespiratory health.

■ You are pleased with how you look. You have enough strength to function well in your daily life of work and recreation, to whatever extreme that may encompass. To remain at

this constant weight, your energy must be in balance:

calories in = calories out

eating = expenditure; exercise

Because expenditure or "calories out" declines with aging (your metabolism slows down and you are less active), a decline in "calories in" (eating less) must accompany the aging processes.

Weight Gain

Weight gain almost always refers to gaining *lean* tissue, or thickening muscle fiber. When you want to look better cosmetically or to increase your strength for a sport or for daily needs, weight training is the type of activity in which to engage. If you are at an overfat weight, in order to simultaneously *gain lean weight and lose extra body fat*, it will require you to eat less while providing the *increased exercise* of weight training. Only if you are at ideal weight or underfat weight should you accompany this weight-gain program with an increase in caloric intake.[2]

Weight gain, then, means increasing muscle mass, or thickening of muscle fibers. You do not gain more muscle cells; you thicken what you presently have.

Weight Loss

Weight loss refers to purposefully losing *fat weight*, never lean weight. Weight loss, of course, can be to both your lean and your fat, according to how you go about losing the weight. Before you spend your money on any unique new weight reduction plan, claim, product, device, or book, call your local Better Business Bureau. If you completely understand the principles of weight loss, you will be able to determine a product's or program's worth before you spend time, money, and energy on it.

Principles of Weight Loss (Fat Loss)

1. *Fat weight is the only kind of weight to lose.* If a product or program claims to "get rid of

excess body fluids," beware! Body fluids are not fat. Unnatural water retention, or edema, is a condition to be monitored and treated by a doctor, not by self-prescribed procedures or products.

2. *If water weight (fluids) is lost by sweating during exercise, it will and should return in 24 hours* to maintain the body's synchronized chemical balance. The energy-producing (metabolic) processes perform best when all of the necessary components are present. Dropping water weight is not effective weight loss. It is part of the fat-free weight and is vital to continuous well-being. You can understand, then why weighing yourself after a strenuous exercise session is an inaccurate time to weigh.

3. *Fat is metabolized more readily and efficiently by performing moderate-intensity exercise for a long time.* If you are able to work continuously at a moderate intensity (lower end of your training zone), for more than 30 minutes, you will tap into the most physiologically sound way to metabolize (burn off) that unwanted body fat. You need to exercise for more than 30 minutes at a time to make significant changes in the fat content of the body.

    Wearing rubber suits, transparent plastic wrap around body parts, or heavy, long-sleeved sweats, nylons, or tights on hot days inhibits the free flow of sweat and does not allow it to perform its function of cooling. In hot and humid settings, wear as little as possible when performing fitness exercises. You cannot metabolize (burn up) fat faster by wearing more clothes.

4. *Fat burns off your body in a general way.* You can't "spot reduce." Spot reducing is perhaps the most prevalent misconception concerning fat weight loss. Many unscrupulous people are defrauding unsuspecting overfat Americans out of millions of dollars every year.

    By your genetic constitution, your body will use up its stored energy (fat) any way it is programmed to do so. You cannot do fifty leg lifts a day and hope to reduce the fat deposits in the area. You will shape up (thicken) the muscle fiber in the area, and toned muscles contain more of the enzymes involved in breaking down fat, but you do not burn off the fat there, or at any specific location. As energy is needed, it is withdrawn first from the immediate sources, and when this is used up, randomly from more permanent storage. It then is converted to an immediate usable form. Thus, at first you may lose weight in places you don't necessarily wish to such as your face or chest/breast area. With perseverance, however, you'll burn off the fat in problem areas, too.

5. *Fat weight loss is accomplished most readily through a combined program of carefully monitoring your food intake and aerobically exercising.* When you monitor food intake (and eat less) and exercise (expend more calories or energy), you lose almost 100 percent fat. This is the only kind of weight that you want to lose. Exercise speeds weight loss, not only by burning calories while you're working out but also by revitalizing your metabolism so you continue to burn calories more readily for the next few hours.

    It is very difficult to lose fat weight by simply eating less food. If you avoid exercise and only choose to severely restrict food intake, when you step on a scale the weight loss is not just fat. According to the way in which you have "dieted," your weight loss is approximately one-half to two-thirds fat loss and *one-third to one-half lean weight loss.* If your lifestyle and habits of eating and exercising don't change after you stop "dieting" and you gain back your lost weight, what you gain back is all fat. You are worse off because you lost both fat and lean and regained only fat. Over a lifetime of "yo-yo" crash dieting, the entire body composition is changing detrimentally.

    There are many ways to *lose* fat weight. Research has determined that the only way to *keep* fat weight off is by having a regular exercise program.[3]

6. *Weight can be both gained and lost through an endurance exercise program.* You will be burning off fat for energy and building up muscle simultaneously. Therefore, if you do not see a change on the scale immediately, don't be disappointed.

7. *A light exercise program tends to increase appetite, and a strenuous exercise program decreases appetite.* After an endurance (aerobic) hour, the desire for food greatly diminishes. You will have time to carefully select or prepare what you know is good for you rather than ravenously grab that easy, high-calorie junk food just sitting around.

8. *Eating less food is easier than exercising it off.* In most high-intensity fitness sessions, you will burn only about 300 calories. If you are seriously interested in losing extra fat weight, think twice about rewarding yourself with high-caloric treats afterward. Instead, replenish your water loss with non-caloric, yet quite filling, ice water.

9. *There is no such thing as a constipated endurance aerobic exerciser or athlete.* Regular, rhythmic stimulation of the entire digestion and elimination processes is one of the side benefits of aerobics.

10. *The body's energy balance determines whether a person gains or loses of body fat.* Proper weight loss is simply the result of taking in less caloric energy and expending more.

WEIGHT-LOSS STRATEGIES

A problem such as being overweight may involve the need for (a) a better self image, (b) a naturally slender eating strategy, (c) learning effective ways to become motivated and make decisions, (d) resolving a phobic response to childhood abuse, (e) learning better social skills, or (f) learning better coping skills.[4]

1 "Naturally Slender" Eating

One of the main differences between naturally slender people and overweight individuals is the construction of their mental images and self-talk concerning food. Overweight people usually construct present-tense pictures and self-talk. They see, smell, hear, experience food, and state internally, "Boy, am I hungry!" The result is that they immediately eat. They focus only on the pleasurable taste of food as they eat.

Naturally thin people usually do not have this present-tense strategy. They create future-tense pictures, self-talk, and feelings. They experience how they'll feel over time.[5] Those future pictures and words help them to master weight management, and they then can enjoy the pleasurable selections they make.

2 Control Panel With One Large Dial

Figure 9.4 was offered to rate the tension and relaxation experienced from stressors. This same type of control panel can be used as an eating strategy. Give each number a rating for how full you feel. Begin with the 5 representing "feeling very comfortable and full," and label in both directions from there. Here are some suggestions for labels, with a corresponding number to get you started, but you should label the control panel the way you want to, according to how you feel.

0-1	Starved/famished
2	The beginning of a meal
3	Only half-full
4	Not quite satisfied
5	**Feeling very comfortable and full**
6	Should have omitted extra helping, or dessert
7	Absolutely stuffed; ate and drank enough for two my size
8	Out of control temporarily
9	Out of control consistently
10	Body is plagued with chronic health risks from long-term overeating.

Then, when selecting and eating food, imagine your control panel and adjust it to how you feel currently, how you choose to feel during the eating process, and how you choose to feel when you're all done eating and drinking.

Caloric Intake and Use

Everything you eat or drink becomes "you" for either a short or a long time. You are what you eat. The food nutrients you eat maintain basic body functions such as breathing, blood circulation, normal body temperature, and growth and repair of all tissue. These are related to fixed factors such as age, body size, and physiological state. Any kind of caloric intake your body doesn't use or doesn't eliminate through solid or liquid waste is kept and worn as body fat for future energy needs.

Caloric Expenditure

Every moment of every day, no matter what activity you engage in, from sleeping to aerobically exercising, you are using up calories. Caloric energy expenditure is influenced most by how physically active you are all day. The body's basic needs are more or less fixed, but the amount of physical exertion is a personal decision.

How physically active your life is depends on your choices of profession and recreational activities. It depends upon a multitude of day-to-day choices: whether to walk to the local store or drive the car; use the stairs or elevator; to rake the leaves or hire it done; go out for a bicycle ride after supper or watch a TV show. How physically active your life is depends as much on attitude as it does on opportunity.[6]

Figuring Weight Maintenance[7]

A. Record your present weight, in pounds.
B. Record your type of lifestyle; number values are:
    12 = sedentary
    15 = active physically

18 = pregnant/nursing
20 = varsity athlete or physical laborer

C. Multiply A times B:

This is your weight maintenance number, or the number of calories per day you need to eat to *stay* at your current weight.

Caloric Expenditures for Various Activities

How many calories you burn per minute during any activity depends upon two criteria:
- *Intensity* (high-, medium-, or low-level work or exercise).
- *Body weight.*

The higher the intensity, the more calories you burn per minute. For example, you expend more energy and calories running a mile than you do walking that mile. The heavier you are, the more calories per minute you will burn (just as full-size cars burn more fuel per mile than small, compact models).

Caloric Intake Needed to Gain Lean Weight

To add one pound of body muscle requires 2,500 calories. (This includes about 600 calories for the muscle and the extra energy needed for exercise to develop the muscle.) Thus, the daily caloric excess, over your maintenance number just figured, is 360.[8] You must be at or below your ideal weight to go on an excess calorie-eating program to gain muscle. You want to use your excess body fat first for your energy requirements.

To gain 1 pound of muscle:
2,500 calories equivalent to 1 pound of muscle
÷ 7 days in a week
= 360 daily excess calories to eat over maintenance intake number

---

Taking in more than 1,000 calories per day over the number needed to maintain weight, however, is likely to result in weight gain as body fat even if you are exercising strenuously on a regular basis.[9]

Caloric Intake Needed to Lose Body Fat

To lose more than two to three pounds of body fat per week is physiologically impossible.[10] Weight loss greater than this represents water and lean body tissue. To systematically drop unwanted extra body fat, you need to drop 3,500 calories a week, or 500 per day, to lose one pound of body fat per week.

To lose 1 pound fat:
3,500 calories
÷ 7 days per week
= 500 calories a day less than your maintenance number

If you desire to drop more pounds per week but the total caloric intake would be less than 1,200, you need to re-establish your goal to lose only one pound per week. You never want to eat fewer than 1,200 calories per day. A daily diet of less than 1,200 calories is likely to be deficient in needed nutrients for you to grow, repair, stay well, and have energy to perform daily tasks and leisure. Sometimes, on a one-to-one basis, a doctor will have a patient eat fewer than 1,200 calories per day, but he or she will provide extensive guidelines and supplementation. This is *only* under the strict supervision of a doctor.

SUMMARY

To maintain a specific weight, caloric input must equal caloric output. To gain or lose weight, there must be an imbalance of energy, regarding your eating and exercising lifestyle habits.

To provide a continual means of self-discipline concerning your weight control:

- Assess your weight whenever your lean or fat weight has increased or decreased substantially.

- Continue setting short- and long-range goals to achieve or maintain an ideal weight;

- Monitor your weight for changes, especially if you are prone to having difficulty in maintaining your weight.

Educating yourself about how to manage your weight can be an interesting experience. It will help you understand how the human body works physiologically and how it doesn't work. You then can be alert to all of the false notions, especially of weight loss, that are rampant today. You can develop a program that will work for you for a lifetime!

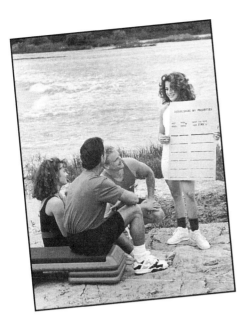

12

Goal-Setting Strategies

Your program is complete. You have learned both physical fitness and mental training strategies on how to become fit and how to maintain that fitness. It's time to plan your future steps and challenge yourself by establishing your priorities, and then setting your program goals. Knowing your priorities will help you to directly establish your goals — the pleasure-filled "ends" you are hoping to achieve regarding your fitness lifestyle.

PRIORITIES

Priorities are the means to reach your goals. They refer to how you spend your time. Make a list of your top ten time priorities — how you *actually* spend your physical and mental energies each week. Rank order them as to which priority is most-to-least important to you. Record any "time-robbers" that take you away from the priority. Can you identify a role model of excellence whom you associate with this priority?

Establishing Priorities

PRIORITIES are the means to your ends. They are things you give TIME to in the wellness areas of your physical/social/emotional/philosophical-spiritual/intellectual/talent expression dimensions.

-1- Top Ten Priorities (Listed In Any Order)	-2- Hours Each Day	-3- Hours Each Week	-4- Time Robbers	-5- Rank Order of Importance	-6- Role Model
•				#	
•				#	
•				#	
•				#	
•				#	
•				#	
•				#	
•				#	
•				#	
•				#	

GOAL-SETTING

Goal-setting requires you to ask yourself a few questions so you can set achievable goals.

1. Ask yourself, *"What will I see, hear, feel in regard to the results?"* You'll recognize these as the components of motivation.

2. Ask yourself, *"Why am I totally committed to achieving each goal?"* Involve your values to answer this question. Values are any of the following: adventure and change, commitment, freedom, pleasure to others, happiness, health, love, power, prestige and worth, security, life purpose, success, talent expression, trust, loyalty.

3. Break the link of the old programmed ways by asking yourself: *"What painful values do I choose to avoid?"* Some of these pain-avoidance values are: anger or resentment, anxiety or worry, boredom, depression, embarrassment, frustration, guilt, humiliation, jealousy, feeling overwhelmed, physical pain, prejudice, rejection, sadness.

4. Re-establish the pleasure link by picturing, hearing, feeling: *"Which actions do I choose to take or do immediately in each goal area*, to master each goal? What is something I can start doing right now and within the next day?"[1]

This goal-setting procedure tells your brain precisely what goal you are choosing to set. It provides solid reasoning for why you're etching this goal-set groove. It also breaks old programming by presenting your pain-avoidance reasons. Last, positive action choices are made immediately to create the motivational pictures, self-talk, and movements necessary to initiate active change in your program. Making an audiotape for yourself by answering the goal questions for each goal you set may prove helpful. You'll find this "blueprinting process" is a unique shortcut to achieving your goals.

Write your responses:

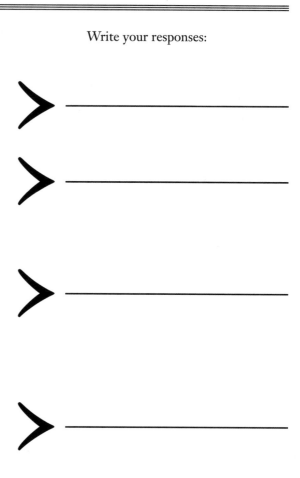

And remember, during this goal-setting process, one end to always keep in mind is to have *fun* during your pursuit of fitness excellence!

SUMMARY

When they are properly internally set and continually nourished, goals will become reality. Believe it and you will see it. Your future resides within you as a rich resource of possibilities.

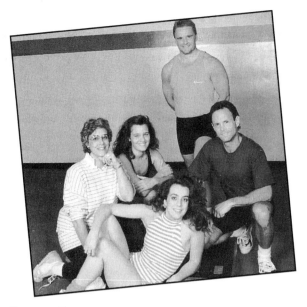

References

Chapter 1

1. Shad Helmstetter, *What To Say When You Talk To Yourself* (New York: Pocket Books, Simon & Schuster, Inc., 1986), pp. 62–71.
2. Hugh Prather, *there is a place where you are not alone* (New York: Doubleday and Company, 1980), p. 96.
3. Quote of Father John Powell SJ, author, from a Personal Wellness course handout of Dr. John Piper, Associate Professor, School HPER, Bowling Green State University, Bowling Green, Ohio.
4. Helmstetter, p. 21.
5. Anthony Robbins, *Unlimited Power* (New York: Fawcett/Columbine, 1986), p. 155.
6. Connirae Andreas, et al., *Heart of The Mind* (Moab,Utah: Real People Press, 1989); Robert Dilts, et al., *Neuro-Linguistic Programming: The Study of the Structure of Subjective Experience* (Cupertino, CA: Meta Publications, 1980); David Gordeon, et al., *The Neuro-Linguistic Programming Home Study Guide* (San Rafael, CA: FuturePace, Inc.)
7. Suzy Prudden, "Affirmations Work!", *IDEA Today*, April 1991, p. 57.
8. Anthony Robbins, *Unlimited Power* (New York: Fawcett Columbine, 1986), p. 31.

Chapter 2

1. Ralph Paffenbarger et al. *New England Journal of Medicine*, 314(10) (March 6, 1986).
2. Kenneth H. Cooper, *Running Without Fear* (New York: M. Evans and Co., 1985), p. 195.
3. Terry W. Parsons, "Positive Lifestyle Strategies," quoting Kenneth Cooper's research, lecture to "Anchor Fitness Course", September 18, 1990.
4. Kenneth H. Cooper, "Run Dick, Run Jane," (Provo, UT: Brigham Young University, 1971) (Film).
5. Kenneth H. Cooper, *The Aerobics Way* (New York: M. Evans and Company, 1977), p. 10.
6. National Vital Statistics Division, National Center for Health Statistics, Rockville, MD, 1988.
7. American College of Sports Medicine 1990: Position Stand, "The Recommended Quality and Quantity of Exercise for Developing and Maintaining Cardiorespiratory and Muscular Fitness in Healthy Adults," *Med. Sci. Sports Exerc.* 22(2), (1990), pp. 265-274.
8. Cooper, "Run Dick, Run Jane".
9. Lenore R. Zohman, et al., *The Cardiologists' Guide to Fitness and Health through Exercise* (New York: Simon and Schuster, 1979), p. 72.
10. *Harvard Medical School Health Letter* Vol. 10(6) (April 1985), p. 3.
11. Ibid.
12. Ibid.
13. ACSM Position Stand, 1990.
14. Ibid.
15. Ibid.
16. Ibid.
17. Ibid.
18. Unpublished research data by Karen S. Mazzeo collected on students enrolled in aerobic dance courses, 1984–1986.
19. G. A. V. Borg, "Psychophysical Bases of Perceived Exertion". *Medicine and Science in Sport and Exercise* 14 (1982).
20. Charlotte A. Williams, "THR Versus RPE. The Debate Over Monitoring Exercise Intensity." *IDEA Today*, April 1991, p. 42.
21. Williams, p. 42.

22. Ken Alan, "A Choreography Primer," *IDEA Today*, January 1989.

23. Lorna Francis, et al., "Moderate-Impact Aerobics." *IDEA Today*, September 1989.

24. Lorna Francis, et al., "Injury Prevention. Low-Impact Aerobics: 'Do's and Don'ts'." *Dance Exercise Today*, Nov./Dec. 1986.

25. Ibid.

26 Alan, "A Choreography Primer."

27. Francis, Lorna et.al. "Moderate-Impact Aerobics." *IDEA Today*, September 1989.

28. Lorna Francis, "Injury Prevention. Combination Aerobics," *Dance Exercise Today*, May 1988.

29. Francis, "Moderate-Impact Aerobics." Also, *Aerobics Choreography* (San Diego: IDEA, Association for Fitness Professionals, 1990).

30. Candace Copeland, *The Low-Impact Challenge for the Fitness Professional* (Newark, N.J.: PPI Entertainment Group/Parade Video, 1991) (Videotape).

31. Francis, "Moderate-Impact Aerobics," 1989.

32. Copeland videotape, 1991.

33. Francis, "Moderate-Impact Aerobics," 1989.

34. Ibid.

35. Ibid.

36. "Research: Caloric Expenditure in LIA vs HIA" from study, 'The Metabolic Cost of Instructor's Low Impact and High Impact Aerobic Dance Sequences.' *IDEA Today*, January 1991, p. 8.

37. "Tempo and Ground Reaction Forces for LIA and HIA," from study 'Comparison of Forces in High and Low Impact Aerobic Dance at Various Tempos,' *IDEA Today*, May 1991, p. 9.

Chapter 3

1. Kenneth H. Cooper, *Running Without Fear* (New York: M. Evans and Company, 1985), p. 128.

2. Ibid, p. 192.

3. Ibid, p. 197.

4. Kenneth H. Cooper, *The Aerobics Program for Total Well Being*. (New York: M. Evans and Company, 1982), p. 141.

5. Lenore R. Zohman, et al., *The Cardiologists' Guide to Fitness and Health Through Exercise* (New York: Simon and Schuster, 1979), p. 87.

Chapter 4

1. Candace Copeland-Brooks, *Moves . . . and More!* (San Diego: IDEA, Inc. 1990) (Videotape).

2. Candace Copeland, *The Low-Impact Challenge For The Fitness Professional*. (Newark, NJ: PPI Entertainment Group/Parade Video, 1991) (Videotape).

3. Julie Moo-Bradley & Jerrie Moo-Thurman, *Aerobics Choreography in Action: The High-Low Impact Advantage*. (San Diego: IDEA, Inc. 1990) (Videotape).

4. Lynne Brick, *Total Body Workout*. (Philadelphia: Creative Instructors Aerobics, 1991) (Videotape).

5. Amy Jones, "Point-Counterpoint. Sequencing a Dance-Exercise Class," *Dance Exercise Today*, May/June 1985.

6. American College of Obstetricians and Gynecologists, *Safety Guidelines for Women Who Exercise* (ACOG Home Exercise Programs) Washington, DC: ACOG, 1986), p. 6.

7. James L. Hesson, *Weight Training For Life* (Englewood, CO: Morton Publishing Company, 1985), p. 33.

8. Ibid.

9. SPRI Products, Inc., 1554 Barclay Blvd., Buffalo Grove, IL 60089. *Pumping Rubber*, (instructions for product use), 1-800-222-7774), 1988.

10. Ibid.

11. Ibid.

12. Ibid.

13. John Patrick O'Shea, *Scientific Principles and Methods of Strength Fitness*, 2nd ed (Reading, MA: Addison-Wesley, 1976), p. 89.

14. Len Kravitz, et al., "Static & PNF Stretches," *IDEA Today*, March 1990.

15. Ibid.

16. Ibid.

17. Ibid.

Chapter 5

1. Joan Price, "Stepping Basics." *IDEA Today*, November/December 1990. p. 57.

2. Len Kravitz, "The Safe Way To Step." *IDEA Today*, April 1991.

3. Sports Step, Inc. *Introduction To Step Training*, (Atlanta: 1989) (Videotape).

4. Lynne Brick, & David Essel, *Pump N' Step*, (1991) (Videotape).

5. Lorna Francis, Peter Francis, and Gin Miller, *Step-Reebok. The First Aerobic Training Workout with Muscle. Instructor Training Manual*. Reebok International Ltd., 1990.

6. Ibid, p. 6.

7. D Stanforth, et al., "The Effect of Bench Height and Rate of Stepping on the Metabolic Cost of Bench Stepping," *Medicine and Science in Sport and Exercise* (abstract), 23 4 (April 1991), S143.

8 Francis, p. 17.

9. Kenneth H. Cooper, *The Aerobics Program for Total Well-Being* (New York: M. Evans and Company, 1982), p. 129.
10. Ibid, p. 144.
11. Level I Walking Only Program was written by Dr. Richard W. Bowers, ACSM-certified Program Director, Fitwell Program, Student Recreation Center, Bowling Green State University, Bowling Green, Ohio. 1990.
12. Kathleen Hargarten, "A Rope-Jumping Class", *IDEA Today*, March 1989.

Chapter 6

1. Lenore Zohman, et al., *The Cardiologists' Guide to Fitness and Health Through Exercise* (New York: Simon and Schuster, 1979), p. 81.
2. Ibid, p. 87.
3 American College of Obstetricians and Gynecologists, *Safety Guidelines for Women Who Exercise* (ACOG Home Exercise Programs No. 2). Washington DC: ACOG, 1986), p. 6.
4. Douglas H. Richie, Jr. "How to Choose Shoes," *IDEA Today*, April 1991, p. 67.
5. Ibid.
6. ACOG, p. 5.
7. Ibid., pp. 4-5.
8. Orthotic for sports shoe prescribed and dispensed by Dr. Charles Marlowe, podiatrist to Karen S. Mazzeo, summer 1983, with accompanying brochure of information.
9. ACOG, No. 2, p. 5.
10. Committee on Nutritional Misinformation, Food and Nutrition Board, National Research Council, National Academy of Sciences, "Water Deprivation and Performance of Athletics." distributed by the Nutritional Education and Training Program, Bowling Green State University, 1981.
11. American Alliance for Health, Physical Education, and Recreation. *Nutrition for Athletes. A Handbook for Coaches.* (Washington, D.C.: AAHPERD, 1971), p. 42.
12. American Alliance for Health, Physical Education, Recreation and Dance. *Nutrition for Sport Success* (Reston, VA: AAHPERD), 1984, p. 2.
13. American College of Sports Medicine. *Encyclopedia of Sports Sciences and Medicine* (New York: Macmillan Company, 1971), p. 215.
14. Ibid, p. 216.
15. American College of Sports Medicine, p. 216.
16. Interview with Jane Steinberg, athletic trainer of intercollegiate sports, Bowling Green State University, Bowling Green, Ohio, Spring 1982.
17. ACOG, p. 6.
18. Interview, Steinberg, 1982.
19. Harvard Medical School Health Letter, Vol. 11, No. 5, p. 4.
20. Len Kravitz and Rich Deivert, "The Safe Way To Step," *IDEA Today*, April 1991, pp. 47–50.

Chapter 7

1. Lorna Francis, Peter Francis, and Gin Miller, *Step-Reebok. The First Aerobic Training Workout with Muscle. Instructor Training Manual.* Reebok International Ltd., 1990.
2. IDEA. *Aerobics Choreography* (San Diego: IDEA: Association for Fitness Professionals, 1989).
3. Ibid.
4. Karen S. Mazzeo, et al., *Aerobic Dance — A Way To Fitness*, 2nd ed. (Englewood, CO: Morton Publishing Company, 1987) p. 112.
5. Ibid, p.113.
6. Francis, et al. pp. 23-25.
7. Ibid.
8. Ibid.
9. Ibid.
10. Ibid.
11. Sports Step, Inc. videotape accompanying The Step, *Introduction to Step Training* (Atlanta, 1989).
12. American College of Sports Medicine: Position Stand, "The Recommended Quality and Quantity of Exercise for Developing and Maintaining Cardiorespiratory and Muscular Fitness in Healthy Adults," *Med. Sci. Sports Exercise* 22:2 (1990), pp. 265–274.
13. Sports Step, videotape.
14. SPRI Products, *Pumping Rubber* (instructions for product use) (Wheeling, IL: SPRI, 1988).
15. Lynn Brick and David Eassel, "Pump N' Step, 1991.
16. SPRI Products, Inc. and Brick Bodies, *Step Strength.* (Wheeling, IL: SPRI Products, Inc.).

Chapter 8

1. Webster's New Twentieth Century Dictionary Unabridged, Second Edition. (New York: Simon and Schuster, 1983) p. 319.
2. Candice Copeland-Brooks, "Smooth Moves," *IDEA Today*. June 1991, p. 34.
3. Joan Price, "Open The Door To Men." *IDEA Today*. February, 1989.
4. Lorna Francis, Peter Francis, Gin. Miller, *Step-Reebok. The First Aerobic Training Workout With Muscle. Instructor Training Manual.* Reebok International Ltd., 1990, p. 6.

Chapter 9

1. Hans Selye, M.D., *Stress without Distress* (Toronto: McClelland and Stewart Limited, 1974), p. 141.
2. Roman G. Carek, Director of the Counseling and Career Development Center, Bowling Green State University, Bowling Green, Ohio, from his Stress Management presentation in the LIFE Seminar Workshop Series, 1982, held at the Student Recreation Center of BGSU.
3. Taken in part from technique developed by Dr. Bernie Rabin, psychologist and lecturer to Karen S. Mazzeo's Personal Wellness, Health Methods, and Stress Management classes 1980–1988, Bowling Green State University, Bowling Green, Ohio.

Chapter 10

1. Nutrition Education Services/Oregon Dairy Council. *"Super Four, A Star-Studded Guide to Food Choices"*, (Portland, 1991).
2. Judy Tillapaugh, "Cross-Training in the Kitchen, " *IDEA Today*, October, 1991, p. 21.
3. U. S. Department of Agriculture, *Food Guide Pyramid, A Guide to Daily Food Choices* (Washington, DC: U.S. Government Printing Office, 1992).
4. National Dairy Council, "Guide to Good Eating: A Recommended Daily Pattern" 4th edition, (B 164-5) (Rosemont, IL: National Dairy Council, 1980). (A revised pamphlet visual is available, "Guide to Good Eating," 5th edition (0001N3) (Rosemont, IL: National Dairy Council, 1991).
5. In-service seminar for Health Education Division Faculty of School of Health, Physical Education, and Recreation, Bowling Green State University. Bowling Green, Ohio, December, 1990, given by nutrition education consultant Jan Meyer of Dairy and Nutrition Council, Mid East, Toledo, OH.
6. Nutrition Education Services/Oregon Dairy Council, "Super FOUR" pamphlet.
7. National Dairy Council, "Guide to Wise Food Choices" (Rosemont, IL: National Diary Council)
8. Wholesome and Hearty Foods, Inc., "Product Line Nutritional Information," given by restaurateur Meredith 'Chip' Myles, Bowling Green, Ohio, spring 1992.
9. Nutrition Education Services/Oregon Dairy Council, "Super FOUR" pamphlet.
10. Jan Lewis, "Nutrition Notes: Nutrition and the Athlete" Workshop Series, Nutrition Education and Training Program, Bowling Green State University, Bowling Green, OH, 1981.
11. U. S. Department of Agriculture, Health and Human Services, Nutrition and Your Health, Dietary Guidelines for Americans" 3d edition, Home and Garden Bulletin No. 232, (Washington, DC: U. S. Government Printing Office, 1990).
12. Lucy M. Williams, lecture and literature, "Shopping Tips For Low Fat, Low Salt, Low Cholesterol Diets," delivered to Karen S. Mazzeo's Anchor Fitness-Personal Excellence class, February, 1991.
13. Ibid.
14. U. S. Department of Agriculture, "Nutrition and Your Health, 1990.

Chapter 11

1. Werner W. K. Hoeger, *Principles & Labs for Physical Fitness & Wellness* (Englewood, CO: Morton Publishing Company, 1991), pp. 80–90.
2. Jan Lewis, "Nutrition Notes. Dietary Guidelines 2," Bowling Green State University, Bowling Green, OH, 1981.
3. Dr. Steven Blair, keynote speaker to the 1992 American Alliance for Health, Physical Education, Recreation, & Dance National Convention, Indianapolis, IN.
4. Connirae Andreas, Steven A. Andreas, *Heart of the Mind* (Moab, UT: Real People Press, 1989), p. 251.
5. Ibid, p. 125.
6. Lewis, p. 6.
7. Kenneth H. Cooper, *The Aerobics Way* (New York: M. Evans and Company, 1977), p. 142.
8. Lewis, p. 4.
9. Ibid.
10. Ibid.

Chapter 12

1. Anthony Robbins, "Personal Power", (Irwindale, CA: Robbins Research International, Guthy-Ranker Corp., 1989. (Audiotape series)

Index